MAD COW DISEASE (BOVINE SPONGIFORM ENCEPHALOPATHY)

Anthrax

Campylobacteriosis

Cholera

Escherichia coli Infections

Gonorrhea

Hepatitis

Herpes

HIV/AIDS

Influenza

Lyme Disease

Mad Cow Disease (Bovine Spongiform Encephalopathy)

Malaria

Meningitis

Mononucleosis

Plague

Polio

SARS

Smallpox

Streptococcus (Group A)

Syphilis

Toxic Shock Syndrome

Tuberculosis

Typhoid Fever

West Nile Virus

DEADLY DISEASES AND EPIDEMICS

MAD COW DISEASE (BOVINE SPONGIFORM ENCEPHALOPATHY)

Carmen Ferreiro

CONSULTING EDITOR
The Late **I. Edward Alcamo**
Distinguished Teaching Professor of Microbiology,
SUNY Farmingdale

FOREWORD BY
David Heymann
World Health Organization

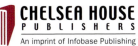

CHELSEA HOUSE
P U B L I S H E R S
An imprint of Infobase Publishing

Dedication

We dedicate the books in the DEADLY DISEASES AND EPIDEMICS series to Ed Alcamo, whose wit, charm, intelligence, and commitment to biology education were second to none.

Mad Cow Disease (Bovine Spongiform Encephalopathy)

Copyright © 2005 by Infobase Publishing

Chelsea House
An imprint of Infobase Publishing
132 West 31st Street
New York NY 10001

ISBN-10: 0-7910-8192-3
ISBN-13: 978-0-7910-8192-1

Library of Congress Cataloging-in-Publication Data
Ferreiro, Carmen.
   Mad cow disease (Bovine Spongiform Encephalopathies)/Carmen Ferreiro.
      p. cm.—(Deadly diseases and epidemics)
Includes bibliographical references and index.
   ISBN 0-7910-8192-3
   1. Prion diseases—Juvenile literature. 2. Bovine spongiform encephalopathy—Juvenile literature. 3. Creutzfeldt-Jakob disease—Juvenile literature. I. Title. II. Series.
RA644.P93F476 2005
616.8'3—dc22   2004024517

Text design by Terry Mallon
Cover design by Keith Trego

Printed in China

Nordica 21C 10 9 8 7 6 5 4 3 2

This book is printed on acid-free paper.

All links and web addresses were checked and verified to be correct at the time of publication. Because of the dynamic nature of the web, some addresses and links may have changed since publication and may no longer be valid.

Table of Contents

Foreword

In the 1960s, many of the infectious diseases that had terrorized generations were tamed. After a century of advances, the leading killers of Americans both young and old were being prevented with new vaccines or cured with new medicines. The risk of death from pneumonia, tuberculosis (TB), meningitis, influenza, whooping cough, and diphtheria declined dramatically. New vaccines lifted the fear that summer would bring polio, and a global campaign was on the verge of eradicating smallpox worldwide. New pesticides like DDT cleared mosquitoes from homes and fields, thus reducing the incidence of malaria, which was present in the southern United States and which remains a leading killer of children worldwide. New technologies produced safe drinking water and removed the risk of cholera and other water-borne diseases. Science seemed unstoppable. Disease seemed destined to all but disappear.

But the euphoria of the 1960s has evaporated.

The microbes fought back. Those causing diseases like TB and malaria evolved resistance to cheap and effective drugs. The mosquito developed the ability to defuse pesticides. New diseases emerged, including AIDS, Legionnaires, and Lyme disease. And diseases which had not been seen in decades re-emerged, as the hantavirus did in the Navajo Nation in 1993. Technology itself actually created new health risks. The global transportation network, for example, meant that diseases like West Nile virus could spread beyond isolated regions and quickly become global threats. Even modern public health protections sometimes failed, as they did in 1993 in Milwaukee, Wisconsin, resulting in 400,000 cases of the digestive system illness cryptosporidiosis. And, more recently, the threat from smallpox, a disease believed to be completely eradicated, has returned along with other potential bioterrorism weapons such as anthrax.

The lesson is that the fight against infectious diseases will never end.

In our constant struggle against disease, we as individuals have a weapon that does not require vaccines or drugs, and that is the warehouse of knowledge. We learn from the history of science that "modern" beliefs can be wrong. In this series of books, for example, you will learn that diseases like syphilis were once thought to be caused by eating potatoes. The invention of the microscope set science on the right path. There are more positive lessons from history. For example, smallpox was eliminated by vaccinating everyone who had come in contact with an infected person. This "ring" approach to smallpox control is still the preferred method for confronting an outbreak, should the disease be intentionally reintroduced.

At the same time, we are constantly adding new drugs, new vaccines, and new information to the warehouse. Recently, the entire human genome was decoded. So too was the genome of the parasite that causes malaria. Perhaps by looking at the microbe and the victim through the lens of genetics we will be able to discover new ways to fight malaria, which remains the leading killer of children in many countries.

Because of advances in our understanding of such diseases as AIDS, entire new classes of anti-retroviral drugs have been developed. But resistance to all these drugs has already been detected, so we know that AIDS drug development must continue.

Education, experimentation, and the discoveries that grow out of them are the best tools to protect health. Opening this book may put you on the path of discovery. I hope so, because new vaccines, new antibiotics, new technologies, and, most importantly, new scientists are needed now more than ever if we are to remain on the winning side of this struggle against microbes.

David Heymann
Executive Director
Communicable Diseases Section
World Health Organization
Geneva, Switzerland

1

Mad Cow Disease: The Beginning

HOLES IN THE BRAIN

Cows are tame, placid animals that eat grass and produce milk and meat. Cows don't normally attack people, stagger as they walk, or kick their owners. Most definitely, cows do not eat other cows. Or so everyone thought until the mid-1980s, in the south of England, when cows started to fall prey to a mysterious illness that turned them into staggering, aggressive animals before it ultimately killed them.

The first documented case of a cow with these unusual symptoms was reported in 1984, three days before Christmas in Sussex County, an hour's drive south of London. According to the animal's owner, this particular cow had refused to go into the milking barn and retreated from contact with other cows. The veterinarian who was called to examine the cow was surprised by these odd symptoms. They were like nothing he had seen before. By the time the cow died in February 1985, other animals at the farm were showing signs of the same illness.

Unable to find an explanation for this strange set of symptoms and thinking the cause could be in the brain, the veterinarian sent the head from one of the cow carcasses (dead bodies) to the Central Veterinary Laboratory (CVL) in Weybridge Surrey for examination. Some sections of the cow's brain had a strange sponge-like appearance under the microscope. Probably thinking that the tissue had been damaged during the preparation of the brain sample, the scientists at CVL did not pursue the matter further.

The mysterious illness continued to spread. Between April 1985 and February 1986, nine cows from the same herd were affected. Soon, cases were reported at other farms. Between December 1986 and May 1987, the same type of sponge-like tissue was discovered in the brains of four cows from three other herds.

In an article published in October 1987, Gerald Wells and his colleagues from the CVL described for the first time the symptoms of the disease in cows and the lesions (abnormal structural changes) in their brains. Specifically, they mentioned finding **vacuoles** (holes) in the gray matter of the brain stem (where the spinal cord joins the brain). These vacuoles gave the brain sections a spongy appearance. It was because of this spongy appearance that they named the disease "bovine spongiform encephalopathy," or BSE (Figure 1.1). In other words, BSE is a disease (pathy) that makes the brain (encephalum) of cows (bovines) look like a sponge (spongiform).[1] The media, however, focused only on some of the more dramatic forms of behavior of the affected cows and dubbed the condition "Mad Cow Disease."

The authors of this first article on BSE also pointed out the similarities between the lesions found in the brains of diseased cows and the lesions that a disease named **scrapie** produced in the brains of sheep.

Scrapie is a fatal nervous system disorder that has affected sheep in England for over 250 years. Yet, scrapie had never been reported in cattle. Scientists believed scrapie was limited to sheep because of what they call the "species barrier." This means that genetic differences between animal species prevent them from passing on a disease from one species to another. The possibility that after all these years, the scrapie agent had changed in some way that allowed it to jump the species barrier and attack cattle was disturbing. This was not only because of the dramatic consequences that a disease like scrapie could have for the cattle industry in the United Kingdom, but

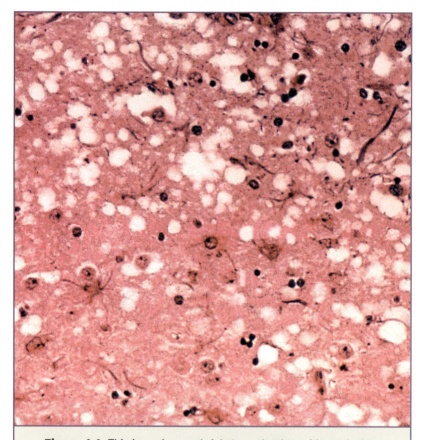

Figure 1.1 This is a micrograph (photograph taken with an electron microscope) of brain tissue from a cow with BSE. The empty spaces are missing brain cells. As the disease progresses, more brain cells die and the number and size of the holes (vacuoles) increase, giving the brain a spongy appearance. This is how the disease gets its name: bovine spongiform encephalopathy (cow with spongy brain disease).

also because the changed or mutated scrapie agent might have acquired the capability of jumping to other species as well. If this were the case, could humans be next?

In December 1986, Raymond Bradley, the department head of the CVL laboratory, wrote to his superiors alerting them to this finding: "The principal lesions," he wrote, "are degenerative and non-specific. If the disease turned out to be bovine scrapie it would have severe repercussions to the export trade and possibly also for humans if for example it was discovered that humans with spongiform encephalopathies had close associations with the cattle."[2]

Bradley's letter eventually reached the Ministry of Agriculture, Fisheries and Food (MAFF), the British equivalent of the U.S. Food and Drug Administration (FDA), and a committee was created to study the disease.

HOW THE COWS WENT MAD

By the end of 1987, 400 cows had been diagnosed with BSE throughout England and Wales, and the number of cases was increasing monthly in what seemed to be exponential growth (rapid multiplication).

To understand how the disease had started and how it was spreading, the MAFF asked John W. Wilesmith, head of the CVL epidemiology department, to conduct a study. Wilesmith gathered data from hundreds of cases and looked for possible causes of the outbreak. The data included details about the animals (such as sex, breed, age, pedigree, origin, identities of the offspring, and dates when symptoms appeared) and about the herds (such as size, proximity to sheep herds in the same and neighboring farms, feeding practices, and types of pharmaceuticals and pesticides used).

The first thing that struck Wilesmith and his team was the fact that, unlike most epidemics that begin with an index case—a first incident of infection—from which the cases spread radially (from a common center), the BSE outbreak had happened almost simultaneously across the United Kingdom. This suggested an infection from a common source rather than one sick animal.

What did all the sick cows have in common? Not much. The cows were of different breeds, had grown up in closed herds in which no new animals had been recently introduced and, in most cases, had not been in contact with scrapie-infected sheep nor with wildlife that might carry disease. Also, the infection didn't follow the calendar year, as it would have if its spread had been associated with the seasonal use of pesticides, vaccines, or herbicides.

The only thing the sick animals had in common was their food. They had all been fed meat-and-bone meal, which was a protein-rich food designed to accelerate their growth and

SYMPTOMS AND OUTCOME OF BSE

BSE develops in cows insidiously, quickly, and relentlessly.

- It is insidious because under apparently mild symptoms lurks a fatal outcome.

- It is quick because the infected cow dies one to six months after the first symptoms.

- It is relentless because there is no cure.

At the beginning of the infection, the cows seem more nervous than usual and have trouble walking. Later, their behavior worsens and they become aggressive and uncooperative, sometimes refusing to be milked and even kicking their owners. They also become increasingly hypersensitive to touch and noise, and their heads may shake in an uncontrollable way. Eventually, the cows' hind legs become so weak that they are unable to stand and they lie down all day, refusing to eat.

Although these symptoms are similar to the symptoms seen in sheep with scrapie, cows don't seem to suffer the severe itching that causes sheep to scratch themselves constantly against fences or walls to the point of losing their fleece.

The media call the cows "crazy" or "mad." But the term *mad* doesn't reflect all the complexity of the symptoms a BSE-infected cow has. A more accurate, but less catchy, description would be "an aggressive, hypersensitive animal that has trouble standing on its hind legs."

increase their milk production. Unknown to most farmers at the time, this **meat-and-bone meal** (**MBM**) was made from the carcasses of dead animals. The feed seemed to be a likely source of contamination. The fact that the number of milk cows falling ill far outnumbered cows grown for meat also pointed to MBM as the source of BSE. Only milk cows are fed MBM. Beef cattle are first fed grass or hay, then fattened with grain.

Still, cows had been eating the meat of other animals in a "human-induced form of cannibalism" for many decades. Why had the disease struck now? Had anything changed in the production of the MBM to explain the sudden outbreak?

RENDERING

Animal parts that humans don't eat and carcasses that are deemed unfit for human consumption (such as those from "downer" farm animals—animals that cannot walk—as well as dead pets and road kill) are transformed into MBM in a process called **rendering**.

Rendering is done by boiling the animal carcasses to separate the fat from the meat. At high temperatures, the fat floats as a creamy white substance called **tallow**, while the heavier protein sinks to the bottom, producing **greaves**, which can be fed to animals. Tallow is used to make candle wax or is mixed with ash and heated again to form soap.

After World War II (1939–1945), tallow was more valuable than greaves, and solvents were added in the process to extract as much fat as possible from the meat. To do this, greaves were crushed and heated to 65° to 70° C (149° to 158° F), and a solvent such as benzene, petroleum spirits, hexane, or perchloroethylene was added. After eight hours, the mixture was passed to another cooker where it was heated to 105° to 120° C (221° to 248° F) for 45 to 60 minutes to vaporize the solvent. After the tallow was recovered, the remaining greaves were blasted with steam for 15 to 30 minutes to remove any residual solvent.[3]

In the late 1970s, the market changed and greaves became more expensive than tallow, and so the solvent extraction process was gradually discontinued. The amount of MBM produced using solvent extraction dropped from about 65% in 1977 to 10% by 1982. At the same time, partly because of the energy crisis of the 1970s and because of a dramatic rise in the price of oil, the duration and temperature of the rendering process decreased.

If, as most experts believe, BSE incubates for three to five years,[4] these two changes in the latter-mentioned process of rendering happened at about the same time that the first cows were getting infected. This means that the rendering changes could be the cause of the BSE outbreak, according to Wilesmith's report of December 1988.

Later experiments showed that exposure to the solvent and higher temperatures did not completely eliminate the BSE agent, but only reduced its infectivity (the capability of causing disease) by a factor of 10. If we also consider that the amount of MBM fed to animals jumped from 1% to 12% during the 1980s,[5] then this increase in infectivity could have been enough to start the outbreak. This is the conclusion reached by a panel of experts led by Gabriel Horn, professor emeritus of zoology at the University of Cambridge, in Cambridge, England, in July 5, 2001, after a thorough investigation of the origins of BSE:

> Rather than switching from a situation where no TSE [transmissible spongiform encephalopathy] infection passed through the rendering system to one where some infectivity passed through and an epidemic ensued, it could be that a threshold level of infectivity was breached. Below this threshold, a certain amount of infectivity survived the rendering process, but not enough to sustain an epidemic; above the threshold (the situation that was perhaps reached after the changes in rendering) enough infectivity survived the

rendering process to initiate and then sustain an epidemic. Such threshold behavior is typical in epidemics of infectious disease.[6]

The fact that MBM is generally produced and distributed locally also supports this theory: Only two rendering plants had continued to use solvent extraction into the 1980s. Both plants were in Scotland, and Scotland was the last region in the United Kingdom to report outbreaks of BSE.[7]

So it seemed certain that the BSE outbreak was an unwanted result of turning cows into carnivores by feeding them MBM. However, scientists were still not sure what specific agent in the MBM was causing the disease.

ORIGIN OF THE BSE AGENT

According to Wilesmith and his colleagues, the agent responsible for causing BSE in cattle was the same that caused scrapie in sheep. In their December 1988 report, they hypothesized that the scrapie agent from sick sheep had remained infectious after the sheep were transformed into MBM by rendering and had finally crossed the species barrier and infected cows. [8]

The sharp increase in the sheep population that the United Kingdom experienced during the 1980s, from 22 million in 1980 to about 35 million by 1988, seems to support this theory. With an estimated 2.25 cases of scrapie per 1,000 sheep, about 80,000 sheep must have been infected in the United Kingdom at the time the first cows became ill. Many of those sheep would have ended up as MBM. [9]

The fact that the outbreak occurred only in Great Britain also pointed to the scrapie agent as the culprit. In the 1980s, Great Britain was the only country that both fed MBM to calves and had scrapie-infected sheep. Other European countries that also had scrapie among their sheep population did not feed MBM to their calves. And, although calves in Australia were fed MBM, Australia's sheep were scrapie-free. [10]

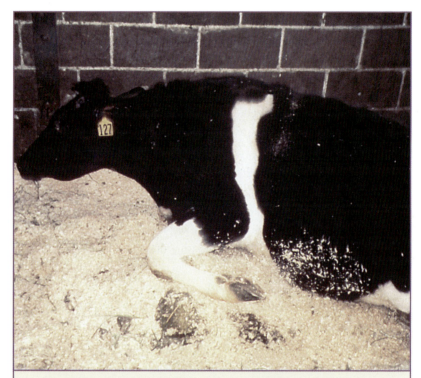

Figure 1.2 During the first stages of the BSE infection, the cows stagger as they walk and become aggressive and antisocial. Eventually, they are unable to walk or even stand and, like the cow shown in this photograph, they just lie down, refusing to eat, until they die.

Not everyone agrees with this theory, however. Richard Lacey of the University of Leeds and Stephen Dealler from Burnley General Hospital, among other researchers in the United Kingdom, believe that the epidemic could have originated with a sporadic case of BSE in cattle. When the sick cow died, the theory goes, the cow was converted into MBM and fed to other cows, thereby spreading the disease (Figure 1.2).[11] Most experts believe this is not a likely scenario. Cows, they argue, do not live long enough to allow a sporadic form of BSE to develop.[12]

Whether the MBM that started the epidemic had been contaminated by a sheep infected with scrapie or by a cow with a sporadic form of BSE is uncertain. What is certain is that contamination of cows from previously infected cows did happen during a second phase of the epidemic,[13] during the years 1985 to 1988, when the carcasses from the early victims of the disease entered the food chain as MBM. Starting in 1989, this second round of infection clearly showed up as an increase in the number of cases of BSE, which occurred after the ban on feeding MBM to cattle had begun.

2

vCJD: The Human BSE

BANS TO STOP THE BSE EPIDEMIC

If MBM were indeed the source of the BSE agent, the first step to halt the epidemic would be to stop feeding the contaminated food to cows. And so in July 1988, the U.K. government, under the recommendations of a committee led by Oxford University zoologist Sir Richard Southwood, issued a ban against feeding ruminant-derived feed to other **ruminants** (hoofed animals including cows, sheep, and goats). A month later, the selling of cows that were obviously sick with BSE as well as the selling of their milk was also banned.

During the months that followed, all cattle suspected of being infected with BSE were slaughtered, doused with gasoline, and burned—to public outcry—in open quarries. Later, as the number of cows and the complaints from neighboring towns grew, the incineration was carried out in enclosed locations. Millions of cows were destroyed in this way.

In February 1989, the Southwood committee presented its final report to the government. The committee supported Wilesmith's hypothesis that the cause of the BSE outbreak had been scrapie-infected sheep included in the MBM fed to cows.

To the knowledge of the committee, scrapie had never infected human beings, and so the report concluded that it is "most unlikely that BSE will have any implication for human health" and also that "the risk of transmission of BSE to humans appears remote."[1] No further measures were recommended, and cows already infected with BSE, but not yet showing symptoms, continued to enter the food chain.

Overall, the report suggested that there were uncertainties in the knowledge of BSE and that if BSE were proved to be more lethal than it seemed at the moment, the consequences could be catastrophic. But the British government ignored the cautionary tone of the report and optimistically concluded that BSE did not pose a threat to humans.

Time would prove the government wrong. But, at the time, any differing opinion in the matter was dismissed as alarmist and ignored.

Eventually, under pressure from the media, MAFF issued a ban in November 1989 on the use of specified bovine offal for human consumption. This offal (waste from butchered animals) included brain, spinal cord, spleen, thymus, intestines, and tonsils—the parts of the animal most likely to be infective. [2]

Meanwhile, the epidemic in cattle continued to spread at an alarming rate. The number of infected cows grew from a few hundred per month in 1988 to more than 3,000 per month in 1992! These numbers didn't start to decline until 1993—later than Southwood's report had estimated. It finally fell to no more than 1,000 per month in 1995 and to about 100 per month in 2000[3] (Figure 2.1). The total number of cows infected with BSE was also much higher than expected: 143,109 cases by February 1995, well over the 20,000 predicted by the committee. The ban, it seemed, was not working as effectively as expected.

One of the reasons why the ban did not effectively slow or stop the epidemic might have been that the British government had not offered adequate compensation to farmers and processors for their losses. At the beginning, farmers were given only 50% of the market value for a cow with BSE. This low price induced some farmers to quickly sell their animals for food at the earliest sign of BSE infection without disclosing the cow's condition. To prevent this, a

Number of cases of bovine spongiform encephalopathy (BSE) reported in the United Kingdom [1]

	ALDERNEY	GREAT BRITAIN	GUERNSEY [3]	ISLE OF MAN [2]	JERSEY	NORTHERN IRELAND	TOTAL UNITED KINGDOM
1987 and before[4]	0	442	4	0	0	0	446
1988[4]	0	2,469	34	6	1	4	2,514
1989	0	7,137	52	6	4	29	7,228
1990	0	14,181	83	22	8	113	14,407
1991	0	25,032	75	67	15	170	25,359
1992	0	36,682	92	109	23	374	37,280
1993	0	34,370	115	111	35	459	35,090
1994	2	23,945	69	55	22	345	24,438
1995	0	14,302	44	33	10	173	14,562
1996	0	8,016	36	11	12	74	8,149
1997	0	4,312	44	9	5	23	4,393
1998	0	3,179	25	5	8	18	3,235
1999	0	2,274	11	3	6	7	2,301
2000	0	1,355	13	0	0	75	1,443
2001	0	1,113	2	0	0	87	1,202
2002	0	1,044	1	0	1	98	1,144
2003	0	549	0	0	0	63	612
2004	0	158	0	0	0	11	169

(1) Cases are shown by year of restriction. Data as of June 30, 2004.

(2) In the Isle of Man BSE is confirmed on the basis of a laboratory examination of tissues for the first case on a farm and thereafter by clinical signs only. However, all cases in animals born after the introduction of the feed ban have been subjected to histopathological/scrapie-associated fibrils analysis. To date, a total of 277 animals have been confirmed on clinical grounds only.

(3) In Guernsey BSE is generally confirmed on the basis of clinical signs only. To date, a total of 600 animals have been confirmed without laboratory examination.

(4) Cases prior to BSE being made notifiable are shown by year of report, apart from cases in Great Britain which are shown by year of clinical onset of disease.

Figure 2.1 As shown above, the number of cases of bovine spongiform encephalopathy (BSE) in the United Kingdom increased from a total of 446 cases up until 1987 to 37,280 in 1992. The number of cases started to decrease in 1993, reaching 2,301 cases in 1999 and 612 in 2003.

100% compensation for BSE-infected cows was offered starting in February 1990.

The situation was even worse in the MBM industry. The plants making MBM were not reimbursed for the product they were supposed to destroy, and either by mistake or fraud, MBM continued to flow into the system and was even used to feed cattle after 1988. In 1996, the government issued a new provision and made it a criminal offense to possess MBM.

Yet, all these measures weren't strict enough or were not taken soon enough, as the emergence of the first human cases of a disease that resembled BSE was about to prove.

CATS WERE NEXT

In May 1990, a cat died after a short illness with symptoms similar to those found in BSE-infected cows. Postmortem examination of its brain indicated that the cat's illness had been caused by a spongiform encephalopathy—a disease until then unknown in cats. In spite of this, the chief veterinary officer, Keith Meldrum, declared on television that there was no cause for alarm. In a letter to the *Veterinary Record*, he wrote, "There is no evidence that the condition is transmissible nor is there any known connection with the other animal encephalopathies."[4] The public thought otherwise.

Fearing that if BSE had been passed to cats through their food, it could also pass to humans through theirs, many people stopped eating beef. The government rushed to reassure the public that humans were not at risk for contracting BSE. To make this point, John S. Gummer, minister of agriculture, appeared on television feeding a hamburger to his four-year-old daughter (Figure 2.2).

Beef was safe, the government insisted. After all, the offal ban was already in effect, and all possible infectious parts of the sick cows had been taken out of the food chain. But had they?

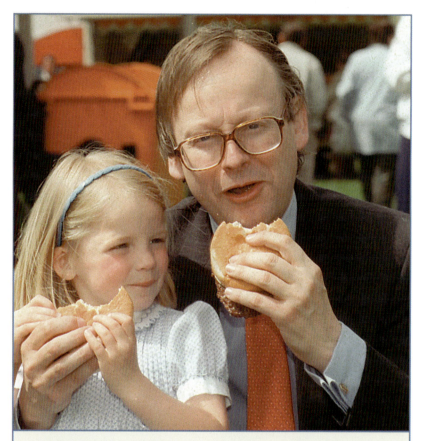

Figure 2.2 This picture was taken on May 16, 1990, when the British minister of agriculture, John S. Gummer, appeared on television eating a hamburger with his daughter. The minister did this to reassure the public that British beef was safe for human consumption.

Leeds physician Richard Lacey didn't think so. In June 1990, he appeared before the British Parliament's Agriculture Committee and declared that meat from BSE-infected animals was still infectious because lymph vessels and nerves, both known to be infectious, thread to muscles and are thus impossible to remove. Since there was no test for BSE, animals that were infected but showed no symptoms could be contaminating the human food supply and would continue to do so unless all infected herds were slaughtered.

Killing millions of cows was not exactly a popular measure. That the government didn't find it necessary to attempt it was not surprising. After all, the government still refused to believe there was any relationship between BSE and the sick cat's death. It was not until four years later, after 62 domestic cats had died, that the government finally admitted that the cats had acquired the disease through pet food contaminated with the BSE agent. Since then, the government has banned specified bovine offal and meat and bone from BSE-suspected cows or cows over 30 months of age from all animal feed.

THE HUMAN BSE

The scientific community considered the possibility that BSE could be transmitted to humans as soon as the disease was identified. An article published in the *British Medical Journal*, back in June 1988, already addressed the question:

> There is no way of telling, which cattle are infected (by BSE) until the features develop, and if transmission has already occurred to man it might be years before affected individuals succumb. [5]

Aware of the possibility that the disease could be in the incubation period (Figure 2.3), a vigilance team had been established to monitor the appearance of any BSE-like case in humans, even before cats had started to be affected. Uncertain of the form BSE would take in humans, the team considered all the cases of Creutzfeldt-Jakob disease (CJD) reported in the United Kingdom. They did so because CJD is a neurological spongiform disease like scrapie and BSE, but CJD affects humans.

The team investigated every single case of CJD, looking for any variation in its pattern: from a change in its symptoms or distribution to an abnormal rise in the number of cases.

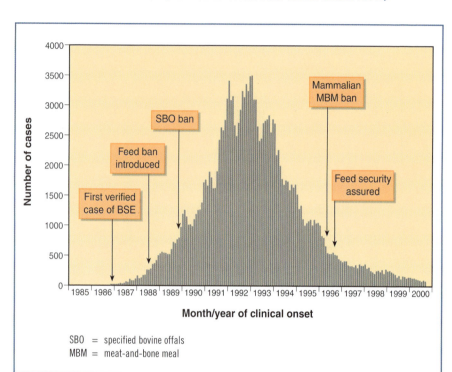

SBO = specified bovine offals
MBM = meat-and-bone meal

Figure 2.3 The graph above represents the course of the BSE epidemic in the United Kingdom from 1986 to 2000. The dates of the major precautionary measures taken by the British government to stop the spread of the epidemic are indicated. Because of the long incubation time of the disease, it took several years for these measures to show their effectiveness.

By the spring of 1996, 10 cases of the 207 cases of CJD that the team investigated presented a new neuropathological (disease in the nervous system) profile (see Chapter 3). This different profile, together with the young age of the victims and the absence of the electroencephalogram (measure of brain waves) features that were typical of CJD, prompted Robert Will[6] and his colleagues to suggest that these cases were a new variant of CJD (nvCJD). This nvCJD, they believed, could be linked to the BSE epidemic in cows. Later, the word *new* was dropped and the disease was named variant CJD or vCJD.

In the mid- to late 1990s, as the theory that vCJD was indeed the human face of BSE, and that humans had contracted it from eating meat or other products from contaminated cattle became accepted, the real "Mad Cow" crisis began in the United Kingdom. Scared of getting infected, people stopped

(continued on page 27)

STEPHEN CHURCHILL: THE HUMAN FACE OF vCJD

Stephen Churchill was 18 years old when he died a frail, mentally incapacitated young man on May 21, 1995.

One of the first victims of vCJD, Churchill's symptoms had started about two years before his death as depression, anxiety, and delusion. According to his sister, he would scream while watching a fire on television, thinking that he was the one burning, or he would believe he was drowning while watching underwater scenes.* Later, he started to react to things that were not even there.

At the same time, Churchill lost interest in life, and his steps became unstable as if he had been drinking alcohol. His condition deteriorated over the following months to the point where he was unable to walk or even to stand. He spent his final days lying in bed or slumped in a wheelchair, unable to talk or even feed himself. Eventually, dementia set in and he became unaware of his surroundings.

After Churchill died of pneumonia, a common fate for victims of neurological disorders, the autopsy of his brain revealed that he had, together with the sponge-like appearance of all CJD victims, the **floral plaques** that came to constitute the trademark of this new fatal disease.

* "The Brain Eater: Mad Cow Disease." *NOVA*. (1998). Produced by Bettina Lerner & Joseph McMasters. Executive Producer Paula S. Apsell. BBC TV/WGBH Boston co-production.

THE FUTURE OF THE vCJD EPIDEMIC

Even though we accept that vCJD stems from the consumption of meat or other products contaminated with the BSE agent, many questions that are critical in determining the course of the BSE epidemic in humans remain unanswered. For instance:

- No one knows why vCJD infects some people but not others who presumably have eaten the same food.

- No one knows the way in which the BSE agent is absorbed. Does it enter the body through the intestines after a meal, or does it enter through cuts or sores in the mouth or fingers of the victims?

- No one knows either the amount of infected beef that needs to be consumed to trigger the disease or whether this amount must be eaten in one single meal or over a longer period of time.

Because the incubation time of BSE in cattle is five years, many infected cows must have entered the food chain before showing symptoms. This makes it difficult to estimate the total amount of contaminated beef that ended up as human food.

The incubation period of BSE in humans is still under debate. Did vCJD patients become infected around 1989 at the peak of the BSE epidemic (which would mean an incubation period of five to six years) or were they infected before, back in 1980, when the first cows were being infected (which would mean an incubation period of 10 to 15 years)?

In spite of such unanswered questions, the future is not that bleak. According to the U.S. Centers for Disease Control and Prevention (CDC), the current risk of contracting vCJD in the United Kingdom is small, or about 1 case per 10 billion servings of beef.[*]

[*]   Yam, P. *The Pathological Protein.* New York: Copernicus Books, 2003, p. 143.

(continued from page 25)

eating British meat. Beef prices plummeted. On March 22, 1996, France declared an embargo (prohibition) on imported beef and live cattle from the United Kingdom. On March 27, the European Union placed a total embargo on all cattle and the products derived from them.

Scientists trying to predict the development of the vCJD epidemic in the United Kingdom had a difficult time. There were so many variables to consider that Oxford University researcher Roy Anderson stated that the number of human cases could reach anywhere between 63,000 and 136,000, whereas a British government study put the high-end figure at 250,000.[7]

By June 2004, only 146 cases of vCJD had been reported by the CJD Surveillance Unit in the United Kingdom[8], but the future extent of the epidemic in humans remains uncertain.

3

Spongiform Encephalopathies in Humans

CREUTZFELDT-JAKOB DISEASE

Creutzfeldt-Jakob disease (CJD) is a progressive neurophysiological disease. Its symptoms are both mental (dementia, psychiatric, and behavioral problems) and physical (muscle twitching and incoordination), and it affects people usually in their mid-40s to late 60s. The condition is named after the two German physicians who first described it.

Although cases of CJD have been described since the 1920s, today it is still difficult to differentiate CJD from other problems such as Alzheimer's disease, multiple sclerosis, and stroke. This is because the symptoms of CJD are not consistent. Not all patients suffer all the symptoms. In addition to the mental and physical symptoms just mentioned, some patients suffer seizures; others go blind.

Laboratory tests do not provide a clear diagnosis of CJD either. Even though the progressive overall deterioration of CJD patients indicates that something is destroying their brain cells, urine tests don't indicate any sign of inflammation or abnormalities in liver function. Blood tests reveal no signs of antibody production that would imply that the body is fighting an infection.

Even the characteristic pattern of periodic spikes that appear in the **electroencephalograms** (tests that register brain waves) of most CJD patients in later disease stages cannot be used as a diagnostic tool either because, again, it doesn't occur in all cases.

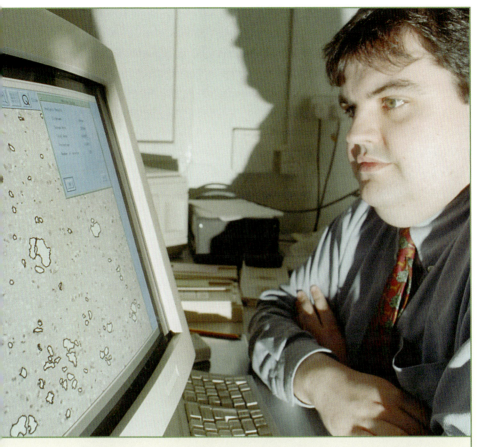

Figure 3.1 A researcher from the CJD Surveillance Unit at the Western General Hospital in Edinburgh examines data on possible cases of vCJD (variant Creutzfeldt-Jakob disease).

The only thing that all CJD patients have in common is the sponge-like appearance of their brain tissue when viewed under a microscope (Figure 3.1). Because of this characteristic, CJD has been included in the group of spongiform encephalopathy diseases.

Because cell structures are mostly colorless, researchers must first dye the samples to be able to see the cells. Using such dyes, researchers have noticed that, in addition to the presence of holes, the brains of CJD patients differ from normal brains in two ways. First, many **neurons** (the functional cells of the brain) are missing. Second, the **glia** (cells that support and protect the neurons) have multiplied, as if trying to fill in the empty space the death of the neurons has left behind. As a result, the samples of brain cells of CJD patients present a star-like appearance because of the increase of astrocytes, the most abundant of the glial cells (Figure 3.2).

In a small percentage (5% to 10%) of all CJD cases, brain samples stained with the dye Congo red show distinct structures, called **amyloid plaques**, which glow green or gold when seen through a polarizing filter.[1] Amyloid plaques were discovered by Robert Koch (1834–1910), while he was examining tissue samples under a light microscope. Koch gave them their name because cross-sections of the tissue samples reminded him of the starch grains found on pears. *Amylum* is the Latin word for "starch."

Amyloid plaques (also called florid plaques due to their appearance) are also present in the brains of people with Alzheimer's and Parkinson's diseases. Unlike the amyloid plaques in the brains of patients with Alzheimer's and Parkinson's disease that are destroyed when treated with **proteases** (active proteins or enzymes that are found in all cells and destroy other proteins), amyloid plaques in CJD cases seem resistant to proteases. This suggests that the amyloid plaques in the brains of Alzheimer's and Parkinson's patients are made of proteins, whereas those in CJD patients are not.

CJD occurs sporadically—meaning randomly and for unknown reasons—at a rate of 1 in 1 million people worldwide, except in Central Africa (which has a low life expectancy of only about 35 years due to the high rate of AIDS infection). Eighty percent of people affected by CJD are between the ages of 50 and 70.[2]

The distribution of CJD in the human population uncannily resembles that of BSE in cows. Why the number of cases of CJD drops among people in their mid-70s is not known.

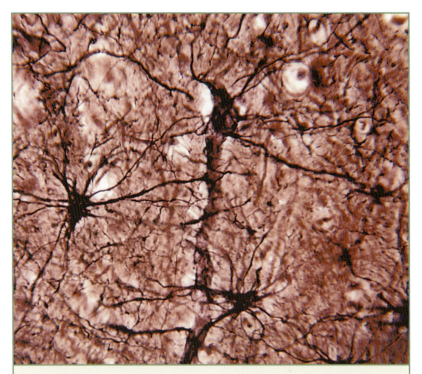

Figure 3.2 The star-like shape of the astrocytes, one of the types of support cells that exist in the brain, are a common feature in micrographs of brain tissue from CJD patients.

SPORADIC OR HEREDITARY CAUSE?

The risk factors that determine whether a person will become affected by CJD are not clear. Some reports indicate that CJD is triggered by an injury or by having surgery with a wound closed with sutures. Others state that having cats or being in contact with certain animals may increase the risk. Still others talk about diet or occupation as the cause. But none of these suggestions has been confirmed as a contributing cause of CJD.

There is one exception: Between 10% and 15% of all CJD cases seem to have a genetic component. If one parent has the disease, the children have a 50% chance of getting it also. This type of CJD, called familial CJD, strikes at a younger age, and its symptoms progress more slowly toward the same fatal outcome.

Other hereditary diseases related to CJD are **fatal familial insomnia (FFI)** and **Gerstmann-Straüssler-Scheinker syndrome (GSS)**. The most characteristic symptoms of FFI

KOCH'S POSTULATES

The German scientist Robert Koch (1834–1910) proposed the following postulates, or steps, which are still followed today when trying to determine the infectious agent of a given disease.[*]

1. Verify the presence of the infectious agent in every case of the disease.

2. Isolate the agent from an infected individual and cultivate it in the laboratory.

3. Inoculate a healthy individual with the laboratory isolate and observe whether the disease is reproduced.

4. Isolate the infectious agent from this second individual. If the infectious agent is the same as the original, repeat inoculation of a healthy individual (second passage) and wait for symptoms of the disease to develop.

Only when the supposed infectious agent complies with these postulates, can it be said that the infectious agent is the cause of the disease.

Because the causative agent of scrapie had not been isolated in the 1930s, these postulates could not be exactly followed then. Yet, the fact that the disease could be reproduced by inoculating healthy sheep with brain tissue from scrapie-infected sheep seemed to indicate that an infectious agent was the cause of the disease, even if the nature of this mysterious agent remained unknown.

[*] Talaro, K., and A. Talaro. *Foundations in Microbiology.* Dubuque, IA: W. C. Brown Publishers, 1993, pp. 355–356.

are insomnia, hallucinations, dream enactments, and twitching. As in CJD, the brains of people who have died of FFI show neuron loss and an increase of glial cells. In this case, the changes are especially severe in the thalamus, the part of the brain that relays sensory signals from the brain stem to areas of the cerebral cortex. In patients in whom the disease lasts longer, the changes also appear in the **cerebral cortex**, a 1/8-inch-thick gray outer layer of the brain that controls higher mental functions.

The first case of GSS was described in 1928 in an Austrian patient. The symptoms of this condition include a gradually worsening imbalance while walking or standing, lack of movement coordination, mood changes that eventually lead to dementia, and a progressive loss of intelligence. Under the microscope, the brains of GSS patients show the typical neuron degeneration with loss of cells, holes, and gliosis (increased production of glia), especially in the **cerebellum** (the part of the brain that governs balance and movement). Also, as in 10% to 15% of sporadic CJD, in GSS cases there is an accumulation of amyloid plaques in the cerebral cortex, the cerebellar cortex, and the basal ganglia. This last characteristic prompted the Austrian neurologist Franz Seitelberger in 1962 to suggest that there was similarity between GSS and another spongiform disease: **kuru** (discussed on page 34).

vCJD

Until 1995, only four teenagers had been diagnosed with CJD during the seven decades that the disease had been known. That was why the appearance of cases of what seemed to be CJD among young people in the United Kingdom gave Robert Will and his team the first indication that they might be dealing with a new disease.

The second clue was the appearance of specific clinical symptoms. These young patients presented psychiatric problems such as depression, anxiety, and delusions in the early stages of the disease before showing the classic symptoms of

CJD, such as dementia and muscle twitching. As in CJD, the outcome of the disease was death, but its progress was slower.

Another difference between classic CJD and this new form was that none of the new patients showed the characteristic pattern of spikes in the electroencephalogram that most CJD patients show in the late stages of the disease. Postmortem examination of the brain tissue of the young victims provided the definitive clue to establish vCJD as a new disease. Samples from the brains of patients with vCJD, like those from CJD victims, showed spongy holes where neurons had died and many astrocytes—signs that the brain was attempting to compensate for the damage. Also consistent with CJD's known targets, these changes had taken place in the hippocampus (the area of the brain that is critical for storing, sorting, and forming memories), the thalamus (the area of the brain that relays sensory signals), and the basal ganglia (the area of the brain that helps control and coordinate movement).

Unlike in CJD samples, all the samples from vCJD patients had amyloid plaques of a very specific nature. These plaques were surrounded by a circle of vacuoles that made them look like a flower (Figure 3.3); hence, the name floral or **florid plaques**. These plaques, very rare in CJD, had been described in samples from the brains of members of the Fore tribe of Papua New Guinea who were sick with still another spongiform disease—kuru—and in the brains of animals with scrapie.

KURU

The Fore called the disease *kuru*, which in their language means "trembling with cold or fear." It described the way the victims shook uncontrollably when they had the disease. News reporters referred to it as the "laughing disease," because the victims seemed to grimace and chuckle for no apparent reason. But kuru was nothing to laugh about. Between 1957 and 1968, it killed more than 1,100 people in a Fore population of 8,000. Its annual death rate of about 1% was 50 times higher

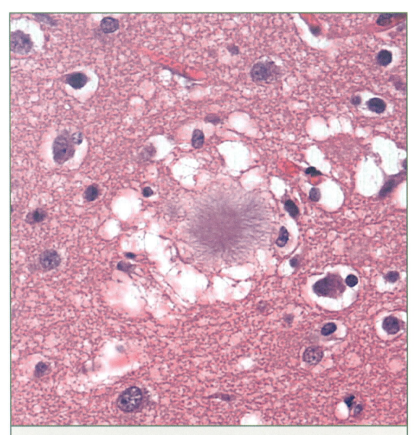

Figure 3.3 Florid plaques appear flower-like, similar to the one seen in this micrograph (center). They have a central core of amyloid surrounded by vacuoles. They are present in brain sections of humans with kuru and vCJD, and of animals with scrapie.

than the death rate from AIDS that the United States suffered in 1995, the peak year of the AIDS epidemic.[3]

Kuru affected the Fore tribe almost exclusively, a primitive people who lived in an isolated region of about 20 by 40 miles in Papua New Guinea (Figure 3.4). Most of its victims were women and children never younger than four years old. Although adult men seemed to be less likely to get kuru, among children, girls and boys were affected equally.

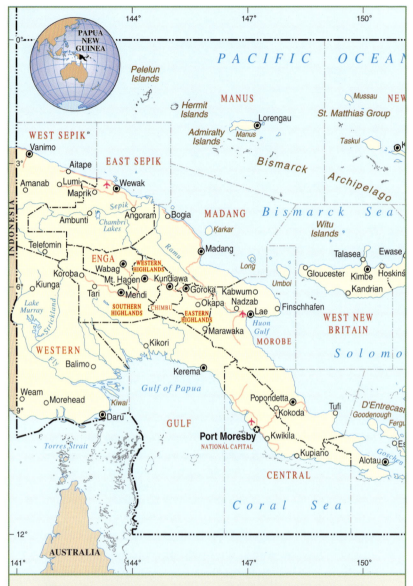

Figure 3.4 Kuru is a spongiform encephalopathy endemic to the Fore, a primitive tribe of the Papua New Guinea highlands, labeled in red at the center of the map. The disease, whose transmission was linked to ritualistic cannibalism among relatives, peaked during the 1950s, and has all but disappeared today.

The symptoms of kuru were consistent. Headaches and pains in the limbs came first. Then, victims developed problems walking and holding their balance and started shaking with spasms. Little by little, they lost control of voluntary movements until they could no longer move or stand. The people affected also developed crossed eyes and emotional instability, and although they seemed to be mentally aware until the end, they were unable to speak. Eventually, they couldn't even swallow and wasted away until they died, usually of pneumonia or other opportunistic infections.

There was no cure for kuru. After the symptoms appeared, adults died in about 12 to 18 months; children in about 3 to 12 months.

Until as late as the 1950s, the Fore still lived in the Stone Age. They had not yet discovered the wheel, and, unaware of metals, they made their tools and weapons from bone or stone. They were cannibals. They ate their dead in a ritualistic feast in which only the family of the deceased participated. Eating the corpse was supposed to give the living the power of the dead person. The Fore didn't eat the bodies of people who had died of known diseases like leprosy, but they did eat the victims of kuru.

For the Fore people, kuru was not considered a disease, but the result of sorcery—a spell that could only be broken by vengeance in the form of a ritual killing called *tukabu*. For each victim of kuru, tukabu was performed on the sorcerer who lived nearby, or if a sorcerer was not found, on a personal enemy or family member. And so, for every death of kuru, another death from tukabu took place.

Vincent Zigas, the first European doctor to reach this isolated region in 1955, didn't believe kuru was caused by sorcery. Zigas first thought kuru could be a degenerative brain disease like Parkinson's, Alzheimer's, or multiple sclerosis. But there was a difference: All these diseases are caused by a pathological alteration in brain tissue, which means that they are not infectious and do not spread or cause epidemics the way kuru was doing.

On the other hand, kuru patients didn't show symptoms of infection either. They had no fever and no sign of inflammation. The results from blood samples sent to the Hall Institute of Medical Research in Melbourne, Australia, to be analyzed came back negative. Scientifically, the cause of kuru was a mystery. Unofficially, however, the consensus was that kuru was being transmitted through the cannibalistic ritual of eating the dead.

As Paul Brown, a Johns Hopkins University resident who joined the research on kuru in the mid-1960s, pointed out,

> Everybody "knew" that cannibalism was the cause of it. It doesn't take a genius, to realize that if you've got a disease reaching epidemic proportions in a group of people that are eating sick people, then a pretty plausible guess is that cannibalism is the cause of the disease.[4]

This theory later proved to be correct, but in 1957, when an American physician named Carleton Gajdusek joined Zigas in his study, the cause of kuru was still elusive. So was the cure. Zigas had tried every drug at his disposal, but nothing had worked.

Thinking that the answers to the mystery of kuru lay in the brain, Zigas and Gajdusek collected tissue samples from the brains of kuru patients and sent them to be analyzed at the National Institutes of Health (NIH) in Bethesda, Maryland. There, a young neuropathologist named Igor Klatzo found extensive neuron degeneration and holes that gave the brain tissue a sponge-like appearance in several parts of the brain, but especially in the cerebellum (not surprisingly, since the cerebellum controls motor functions such as walking).

The holes in the brain reminded Klatzo of the features of an obscure disease he had studied during his medical training—Creutzfeldt-Jakob disease. Still, there were differences:

75% of the kuru samples had knots of proteins, also called amyloid plaques. These plaques, which were similar to the amyloid plaques seen in other degenerative diseases such as Alzheimer's, were not usually present in CJD patients.

Besides, the fact that kuru targeted mainly women and children, whereas CJD was a disease of middle and old age, the epidemic way in which kuru spread, and the differences in symptoms suggested that CJD and kuru were not the same disease.

In 1959, as part of a traveling show about his research in kuru, Gajdusek brought Klatzo's photographs to London. It was there that William J. Hadlow, a young American veterinarian, saw them. Hadlow was shocked by the pathological changes kuru caused in the brain tissues. He had seen these changes before, not in humans, but in the brains of sheep affected by another mysterious disease—scrapie.[5]

4

Scrapie and Other Spongiform Encephalopathies in Animals

A HISTORY OF SCRAPIE

Scrapie is a fatal illness in sheep, which has been known in Europe for over 250 years. It prompts sheep to scratch themselves furiously against walls and fences as if suffering extreme itching. Yet, upon examination, their skin shows no signs of irritation.

First described in England in 1732, scrapie was then known as rickets ("shaking"). It was soon reported in Germany (1759) and then throughout the rest of Europe. By the beginning of the 20th century, it had become endemic (permanent) in England, where it affected 1% of adult sheep annually. It came to the United States in 1947, and today exists in all sheep-raising countries with the exception of New Zealand and Australia.

The following sentence from an 18th-century report from Germany describes quite accurately the symptoms of the disease: "[Animals suffering from scrapie] lie down, bite at their feet and legs, rub their back against posts, fail to thrive, stop feeding, and finally become lame."[1]

Scrapie progresses quickly from early symptoms (scratching, running wildly, shivering, and an avoidance of the rest of the flock) to the more severe (pronounced shaking of the head and muscles, lack of coordination, loss of appetite, rubbing flanks to the point of damaging the skin, showing an awkward gait while walking as if the forelegs were trotting and the hind legs galloping, and a tendency to fall). In the last stages of the disease, the affected sheep stagger as if drunk and finally just lie down, emaciated, unable to drink or eat. Never in the course of the disease does the animal show any fever.

Although the symptoms of scrapie suggested a brain degenerative disease, the brain from a scrapie-infected sheep was no different from that of a healthy sheep, at least to the naked eye.

But when, in 1898, French veterinarian Charles Besnoit examined samples from the brains of sheep that had died from scrapie under the microscope, he found bubble-like vacuoles (holes) in the spinal cord and peripheral nerves. These vacuoles were so widespread in the brains of scrapie-affected sheep that the identification of spongiform degeneration (holes) in the cerebellum of a sheep became the diagnostic indicator of scrapie.

In the 1950s, American veterinarian William Hadlow, who was working at Compton Laboratory in the United Kingdom, found that these holes existed not only in the cerebellum, but also in the cerebral cortex. He found that the nerve cells were shrunken and that there was an abnormal multiplication of astrocytes, which support the neurons in the brain.

Scrapie is always fatal. Once a sheep show signs of the disease, death follows in a matter of months (anywhere from six weeks to six months). "The best solution, therefore," the German veterinarian J. G. Leopold advised back in 1759, "is to dispose of it [the affected sheep] quickly and slaughter it away from the manorial lands, for consumption by the servants of the nobleman."[2]

Despite the killing of sick animals and even the later, more drastic, measures of mass slaughtering of all the animals that might have been exposed to the disease, scrapie had not been eradicated. If New Zealand and Australia are scrapie-free, it is only because the disease has never been introduced into these countries. When, in 1952, some cases of scrapie were found in Australia in a newly imported group of sheep, the whole group was promptly isolated and killed.

ONE DISEASE; MANY NAMES

The name *scrapie* comes from the verb "to scrape," and refers to the way affected sheep rub themselves raw as if suffering an unbearable itching. In Spain, the current name of the disease, *prurigo lumbar*, also refers to this itching. *Prurigo* means any kind of irritation of the skin. Yet, through the two and a half centuries since its discovery, scrapie has been known by other names.

When first reported in England in 1732, it was called "rickets" or "shaking," the name emphasizing, this time, the incontrollable shaking of the head and other muscles of affected animals. The modern term for the disease in French, *la tremblante*, has this same meaning.

Other names of the disease reflect its neurological symptoms. That is the case of the French terms *maladie folle* and *maladie convulsive* (the disease of madness and convulsions), *maladie nervese* (nervous disease), *nevralgie lombaire* (lumbar neuralgia), and *vertige du mouton* (sheep dizziness).

Finally, the French also use the term *maladie chancelant* (wobbling) and the Germans called the disease *Traberkrankheit* (*Traber* means "trot"), referring to the awkward gait of the affected animals.

The disease has so many different names because it seems to have been discovered and forgotten several times. Two factors may have contributed to this: One is that the farmers, aware that any case of scrapie among their sheep would make the entire flock suspicious and thus lower its price, may have hidden the fact that any of their sheep had scrapie. The second factor was that the disease sometimes lies latent for years, before resurfacing again.

The persistence of scrapie in an area where it has been reported is remarkable. For instance, in 1946, in Iceland, all flocks with cases of scrapie among their sheep were slaughtered and their pastures burnt and left empty for up to three years. Still, scrapie resurfaced within four years after sheep from scrapie-free flocks were reintroduced into those areas.

HEREDITARY OR INFECTIOUS CAUSE?

From the beginning, whether scrapie was hereditary (caused by a defective gene passed from a ram or ewe to its offspring) or transmitted from sheep to sheep (horizontal transmission) by an infectious agent was not clear. In fact, the data on scrapie were so peculiar and contradictory that some people claimed it was both infectious and hereditary, even though no disease has ever been found to be so.

Reverend Thomas Comber, one of the first to report on scrapie, wrote in 1772: "I do not find, Sir, that this Distemper is infectious: but alas! It is hereditary, and equally from Sire and Dam, and like other hereditary Distempers, may lie latent one Generation . . . and then revives with all its former fury."[3] Back then, many farmers shared his belief, having observed that in a given flock, only the offspring of certain rams were affected by scrapie.

Yet sometimes scrapie seems to pass from sheep to sheep within a flock, which suggests that scrapie is contagious. This belief prompted the German veterinarian J. G. Leopold, writing in 1759, to suggest that any animal suffering from scrapie should be quickly isolated and slaughtered to avoid infecting the remainder of the flock. However, if scrapie is contagious, why do sick and healthy sheep sometimes live together and even rub against one another without passing on the disease? Besides, an infectious disease would result in fever as the body of the infected animal reacts to the foreign agent. Yet, scrapie-infected sheep never show any fever.

Other causes of scrapie have been suggested over the years. Some, like linking scrapie to environmental factors, diet, or the conditions in which the animals breed, were plausible; even if further experiments have not supported them. Others were downright outrageous, like the 18th-century suggestions that scrapie was caused by an excess of sexual ardor in rams, by loud thunder, by the sheep being chased by dogs, or by the sheep being exposed to bright sunshine during the first few days after shearing.

The contagious nature of scrapie was established in 1936 when healthy sheep developed the disease after being inoculated with extracts from the brains of affected sheep. Yet, the question of how scrapie was transmitted in nature continued to puzzle scientists well into the 20th century.

In the 1970s, Iain Pattison and his colleagues at the British Agricultural Research Council's Institute in Compton, working under the premise that scrapie was transmitted orally, fed sheep different parts of infected animals and waited for the disease to develop. The conclusion of their experiments, published in 1972, was that scrapie was transmitted by eating the **placenta** of infected sheep. (The placenta is the organ that unites mother and offspring during pregnancy and is expelled at birth.) The fact that sheep are kept together during lambing and all of them share in the eating of the placentas expelled after the birth of lambs seems to support this theory.

This theory also explains the observations recorded by Icelandic researcher Bjorn Sigurdsson in 1954, that when a flock of healthy animals is reintroduced in a field where scrapie-infected sheep have lived, the sheep eventually come down with scrapie. On the other hand, a healthy flock kept in a field where no infected sheep had ever lived remains healthy. Seemingly, the scrapie agent from contaminated placenta is able to survive in the soil where infected sheep once grazed.

Despite these experiments and the ones on transmissibility, as late as 1998, some scrapie specialists[4] still defended the notion that scrapie is exclusively a hereditary disease.

SCRAPIE PROVES TO BE TRANSMISSIBLE

If scrapie is caused by an infectious agent, then inoculating healthy sheep with infected tissue should reproduce the disease. Yet, early attempts to transmit scrapie this way were unsuccessful.

Finally, in 1936, two French veterinarians, Jean Cuille and Paul-Louis Chelle, injected a homogenate (tissue that has been homogenized—that is, blended into a uniform mixture) of spinal cord from a scrapie-infected sheep into the eye of a healthy one and waited for the sheep to develop the disease. They waited for a much longer time than any of their predecessors had ever waited. Fifteen months later, their patience was rewarded when the inoculated sheep showed symptoms of scrapie.

They repeated the experiment, this time by injecting infected tissue into the brain or under the skin of healthy sheep. With an incubation time that varied between one year (in the case of injection to the brain) and two years (for inoculation under the skin), 25% of the sheep came down with scrapie as well. In 1939, they also reported that they had transmitted scrapie to goats. Transmission occurred in 100% of goats, and the incubation time was 25 months.

Because so many researchers had failed to transmit scrapie, Cuille and Chelle's success was met with skepticism. But soon their results were confirmed in an unexpected way. In the 1930s, about the same time that Cuille and Chelle were doing their experiments on the transmissibility of scrapie, Dr. William Gordon and his colleagues at the research facility in Compton were working on a vaccine to protect against another sheep disease. The disease, called **louping ill** or **loup**, is caused by a tick-borne virus that induces brain damage in sheep. To make the vaccine, the scientists homogenized brain, spinal cord, and spleen tissue from sheep that were sick with louping ill. After diluting the sample with saline solution, they added formalin (a solution of formaldehyde) to inactivate the virus. This would make the virus unable to cause an infection, yet still allow it to trigger the defense mechanism in the sheep's body (by activating its immune system). Inoculation with the inactivated virus would protect the sheep from infection if, at a later occasion, it was exposed to the active virus.

Dr. Gordon and colleagues produced several batches of vaccine during the years 1935 and 1936, which they used to inoculate sheep at risk. The vaccine worked, and the sheep did not develop loup. But, to the researchers' horror, some of the sheep inoculated with the batch made in 1935 showed symptoms of scrapie two and a half years after vaccination. When they checked the records of the sheep used that year to prepare the vaccine, they realized that some of the sheep had been in contact with sheep that had later developed scrapie. So it seemed that, unknown to the experimenters, the loup vaccine had been contaminated with the scrapie agent.[5]

This unwanted result of the loup vaccination program confirmed that scrapie was transmissible. It also revealed that the scrapie agent was resistant to formaldehyde—a very unusual characteristic for an infectious agent and one that no known virus or bacterium shares.

TRANSMISSIBLE MINK ENCEPHALOPATHY

Spongiform diseases have been described in humans (CJD and kuru); cats, sheep, and goats (scrapie); and cattle (BSE or Mad Cow Disease). Another lethal disease with symptoms of neurological degeneration (including aggressiveness, incoordination, and self-mutilation) and similar pathology of microscopic holes in the brain of its victims was reported in the United States in 1947, 1961, 1963, and 1985 among minks raised on farms.

Like scrapie, the mink disease was transmitted by inoculating infected brain tissue into the brains of healthy animals and was thus termed **transmissible mink encephalopathy**, or TME. The effects of TME on a mink ranch were devastating. In 1947, 1,200 minks died in the outbreak. In 1961, 20% to 30% of the affected mink herds died. In 1963, the mortality among the adult animals of the affected herd was a striking 100%, whereas, in 1985, TME killed 60% of the 7,300 minks in five months.

Given the similarities between TME and scrapie, researchers turned to scrapie for clues on how the TME outbreaks had started. Scrapie was transmitted among sheep by eating infected placenta. Minks do not eat placentas, but, being carnivores in the wild, when kept on farms, they are fed raw meat, fish, offal, cereal, and meat-and-bone meal (MBM) produced after the rendering of slaughtered animals. Could it be that some scrapie-infected sheep had been accidentally included in the minks' food? If so, was eating scrapie-infected sheep the cause of the TME outbreak? It was a likely possibility. However, when Richard Marsh, a researcher at the University of Wisconsin–Madison, tried to infect minks with brain tissue from scrapie-infected sheep, the results didn't seem to support this theory. Although healthy minks inoculated with infected mink brain showed symptoms of the disease in 7 to 12 months, minks inoculated with scrapie-infected brain tissue didn't start to show symptoms until after 12 months. And Marsh couldn't get any infection by feeding the infected sheep to the minks.

Besides, the first TME outbreak had occurred in Wisconsin in 1947, before the arrival of scrapie to that state. Furthermore, neither sheep remains nor feed supplements of MBM were fed to the minks affected by TME in the 1985 outbreak at another ranch in Wisconsin. However, the minks *were* fed sick and downed cows that the farmer collected within a 50-mile radius of his ranch. Because the first cases of BSE were being discovered in the United Kingdom in 1985, Marsh immediately wondered whether a cow harboring BSE or a similar disease had been the cause of the outbreak.

Because any remains of the suspected cows were gone by the time Marsh arrived at the farm, he had to go the long way to check his theory. He first inoculated two young bulls with infected mink brain. When the steers collapsed and died eight to nine months later, he used their brains to either inoculate or feed healthy minks. The minks were dead in four months when inoculated, and seven months when they had acquired the disease by eating the contaminated brains.

The quick appearance of the disease in minks implied that there was no species barrier between mink and cattle. This supported the theory that minks had contracted TME from cows.

Further experiments confirmed Marsh's results. In 1990, William Hadlow—the scrapie expert who had first suggested that kuru and scrapie could be related—succeeded in infecting steers with brains from TME-infected minks that had been stored frozen since the 1963 outbreak. Under the microscope, the steers' brains had the typical spongiform appearance. Yet, the symptoms of the disease and the areas in the brain affected were different from the ones BSE was causing in British cows. Moreover, when minks were inoculated with brains from BSE-infected cows, they developed a TME-like disease that was similar but not identical to TME.

For Marsh and Hadlow, the conclusion was unavoidable: Minks had acquired the disease from cattle affected by a spongiform-like disease that was not BSE. They concluded: "If TME results from feeding infected cattle tissues to mink, there must be an unrecognized BSE-like infection in American cattle and in other countries where TME has been reported." (Isolated TME outbreaks had also occurred in Finland, Russia, and Germany).[6]

Because downed and sick cows were still being used at the time in the United States to feed cattle, Marsh was worried that the American strain of BSE could be amplified by this process and provoke an epidemic similar to the one BSE was causing in the United Kingdom. Marsh lobbied hard to end the practice of using sick cows in feed against great opposition, especially from the powerful rendering industry. Finally, in 1997, shortly after Marsh died, the FDA approved the ban on rendering cattle into cattle feed in the United States.

CHRONIC WASTING DISEASE IN ELK AND DEER

The possibility of spongiform diseases occurring spontaneously is not so far-fetched. After all, CJD does occur sporadically in 1 in 1 million humans, and a French veterinarian had already described what he called "a case of scrapie in an ox" as far back as 1883. An 18th-century English veterinarian also described symptoms similar to scrapie in a deer kept in a park. So, for Joe Gibbs, a researcher of viruses and an expert on kuru, the discovery of another spongiform encephalopathy disease affecting mule deer and elk in the United States was not surprising.[7]

The first case of what is now called **chronic wasting disease** (**CWD**) was reported in a captive mule deer at the Colorado Foothills Wildlife Research Facility in 1967. Between 1967 and 1979, the disease killed 53 mule deer and one black-tailed deer; this translates to 90% of the deer that stayed at the facility for more than two years.

Then, in 1980, cases of CWD appeared at the Sybille Research Unit in Wyoming. Although situated 120 miles northwest of the Colorado Foothills Wildlife Research Facility, both units had shared deer. This suggested that CWD was being transmitted horizontally from deer to deer. Soon, cases were also reported among elks at both facilities. Deer affected by CWD develop a blank stare, start to drool and slobber, and walk in repetitive patterns while their bodies waste away. They die in about three to four months after the onset of symptoms (Figure 4.1). How CWD originated remains a mystery, as is the way it spreads from animal to animal, although it has been suggested it could be passed through contact with the saliva or urine of infected animals.

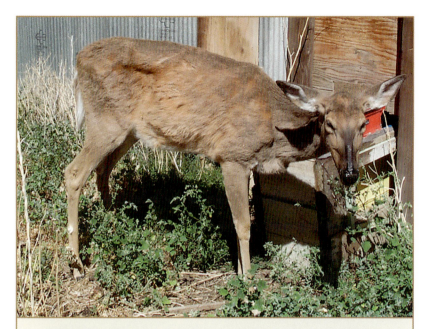

Figure 4.1 The deer in the above photograph suffers from chronic wasting disease (CWD). CWD is a transmissible spongiform encephalopathy, similar to BSE and scrapie, that affects deer and elk. No evidence has been found to date that CWD can be spread to humans who eat the infected meat of these animals.

At first, CWD was thought to be a result of nutritional deficiencies or poisoning, or even stress. But in 1977, Elizabeth S. Williams at Colorado State University found microscopic holes in the brain tissue of infected deer and realized that CWD was a spongiform encephalopathy.[8]

For almost four decades, CWD was confined to a 15,000-square-mile area in northeastern Colorado and southwestern Wyoming and Nebraska around the two facilities mentioned above. However, since 1996, a second epidemic has appeared among elk herds that were kept for meat and antlers in small ranches. (Antlers are sold as a supplement in vitamin stores and as an aphrodisiac in Asia.) The ranches are scattered across six states in the United States (Colorado, Kansas, Montana,

Nebraska, Oklahoma, and South Dakota) and two Canadian provinces. The affected animals were probably transported by truck from the contaminated areas while still incubating the disease: It takes about 20 to 30 months for symptoms to show. Again, the disease also spilled from the ranches into the local population of wild deer in the states already mentioned, plus New Mexico and Minnesota.

Whether as a consequence of the relocation of diseased animals from affected areas or by other unknown means, CWD has also spread across the Mississippi River into the free-ranging white-tailed deer in Wisconsin and Illinois.

Over the years, several attempts have been made to eradicate CWD. At both the Sybille and Fort Collins, Colorado, facilities, researchers killed all the deer and elk in the main area. Even after repeatedly spraying the area with chlorine, the disease returned after the deer and elk were reintroduced one year later.

In Wisconsin, the Department of Natural Resources started a campaign of massive killings in June 2002, with the goal of eliminating 25,000 deer in a 411-square-mile zone, 40 miles west of Madison, Wisconsin. By the end of 2003, they had found 50 sick deer among those killed. Yet, in January 2003, infected deer were found among those killed by hunters outside the eradication area. Whether CWD can infect humans is not known. Three cases of young patients who had contracted CJD and also had regularly eaten venison (meat of deer, elk, and other game animals) have been reported since 1997. But on further investigation, the Centers for Disease Control and Prevention did not find a link between the deaths of these young people and CWD.

CWD could also pose a threat to humans by passing the disease to domestic livestock first. Experiments are under way to assess whether this is possible. Nevertheless, since November 2002, the FDA has forbidden the rendering of suspected CWD deer into animal feed.

5

Spongiform Encephalopathies Are Transmissible

EXPERIMENTS ON TRANSMISSION

In 1959, after seeing the pictures Gajdusek had brought to London to document his discoveries on kuru (see Chapter 3), Hadlow wrote a letter to the *Lancet*, a prestigious British medical journal, comparing kuru with scrapie. This letter marked the first time that scrapie, an illness that affects only animals, was mentioned in a medical publication. Hadlow highlighted the striking similarities between kuru and scrapie: Both diseases were endemic (permanent) in certain populations, where they occurred in only about 1% of individuals (sheep or humans) and could be introduced in a previously healthy group by the transfer of one individual from an affected group. Both kuru and scrapie developed without fever or signs of infection and were fatal within three to six months from the onset of symptoms. The symptoms of scrapie and kuru were also similar: loss of coordination, tremors, and changes in behavior—changes found in the brains of victims, nerve degeneration that would cause the typical spongiform appearance under the microscope, astrocyte formation, and lack of inflammation.

By the time Hadlow wrote this letter, experiments of transmissibility had already been successfully completed with scrapie, but not with kuru. It was obvious to Hadlow that if both diseases were so similar, then kuru was also likely to be transmissible. At the end of his letter, Hadlow suggested to Gajdusek that it would be worthwhile to try to inoculate brain tissue from kuru patients into healthy brains—not of humans, of course, but of their closest relatives, primates.

Gajdusek had never heard of scrapie and believed kuru was hereditary, but he took the letter seriously. He went to Europe and learned about scrapie from experts at Compton Laboratory in Edinburgh, Scotland; and Iceland. Although convinced of the need to perform the experiments of transmission, Gadjusek was unwilling to leave the freedom of the New Zealand highlands and wait for months or maybe even years for the inoculated animals to come down with the disease. He tried to recruit Hadlow to monitor the inoculation of the primates, but Hadlow declined. Finally, Gajdusek convinced a virologist (scientist who studies viruses), Clarence J. "Joe" Gibbs, to remain at the facility that the NIH had provided in the Patuxent Wildlife Research Center in Laurel, Maryland, and perform the experiments.

In August 1963, the inoculation of primates and other mammals with kuru-infected brains began. "By the end of 1963," Gibbs recalled, "I had inoculated about 10,000 mice, 7 chimpanzees, and 75 smaller non-human primates."[1]

In June 1965, one of the chimpanzees came down with the "shakes." Soon, two others followed. The animals deteriorated rapidly, showing clear symptoms of neuron degeneration. The first chimpanzee was sacrificed in October 1965. Under the microscope, the chimpanzee's brain looked exactly like the brains of the human victims of kuru. As Hadlow had predicted in 1959, kuru was transmissible.

Gajdusek, Gibbs, and Michael Alpers—a doctor who had joined Gajdusek in New Zealand—confirmed this result by successfully transmitting kuru from these first chimps to several other chimpanzees: following the second of Koch's postulates (see box on page 32). The incubation period of the disease in this second passage (infection of a chimpanzee with an inoculum from a sick chimpanzee) fell to one year, showing that the infectious agent was adapting to its new host. Gajdusek expanded the goal of his research to include other chronic nervous system diseases such as multiple sclerosis, amyotrophic lateral sclerosis, Parkinson's disease, and CJD. Only CJD proved to be transmissible (in 1968) with an incubation period for chimps of 10 to 14 months. The incubation period for kuru was longer, 14 to 39 months.

Over the next years, in the late 1960s, Gajdusek and Gibbs transmitted kuru, CJD, scrapie, and TME with various levels of success to chimpanzees, gibbons, different types of monkeys, sheep, goats, calves, mink, albino and black ferrets, cats, raccoons, skunks, mice, rats, hamsters, gerbils, voles, guinea pigs, and rabbits.

Although the symptoms and other features of all human neurodegenerative diseases typically overlap, only kuru and CJD share both the property of being transmissible under laboratory conditions and the progressive vacuolation—that is, the appearance of holes within the neurons, which eventually leads to neuron destruction.[2] Because of these properties, CJD and kuru, together with similar diseases in animals, are referred to as "transmissible spongiform encephalopathies" or TSEs.

IATROGENIC TRANSMISSION

The fact that CJD could be transmitted to animals raised the question of whether it could also be spread to humans. It was a likely possibility, and a scary possibility as well, because it opened the door for **iatrogenic transmission**, the spread of a disease by accident in a medical setting.

Could humans get infected with CJD through contact with contaminated surgical or medical equipment? Could they get infected when receiving organs or hormone preparations from an infected CJD victim with no symptoms? These are questions scientists should have asked themselves at the time, which might have prevented iatrogenic transmission of CJD from occurring. Yet, CJD is such a rare disease (it affects just 1 out of 1 million persons worldwide), and, back in the 1960s, it was such a little-known disease among physicians that the questions were never properly addressed, and no measures were taken to prevent the risk.

In 1976, a woman in the United States who had received a cornea transplant died of CJD. It was also in 1976 when Alan Dickinson, a scrapie researcher from Compton Laboratory in Edinburgh, realized that the way laboratories worldwide were obtaining growth hormone from the pituitary glands (small, two-lobed glands connected by a thin stalk at the base of the brain) of cadavers (dead bodies) was concentrating the CJD agent. At the time, the growth hormone was injected into children as a treatment for dwarfism.

Hormones are chemical messengers that play an essential role in the development of the human body. They are secreted by endocrine glands and transported by the bloodstream to their target cells. Once bound to their target cells, the hormone sets in motion (in fact, the Greek word *hormaein* means "to set in motion") a biochemical reaction that allows the target cells to carry out their function. In the case of growth hormone, it allows the body to grow normally.

Growth hormone is a protein that is made in the pituitary gland. Isolated in the 1950s, growth hormone has been used since 1959 to help increase the height of children who suffer from dwarfism.

As Dickinson realized back in 1976, if one of the pituitary glands used to extract the hormone came from a CJD victim, the whole batch would be contaminated and would put thousands of children at risk.

Dickinson alerted the British Medical Research Council (MRC) to this possibility, and, in turn, the MRC commissioned Dickinson to test his hypothesis. So Dickinson designed an experiment. He injected mice with human growth hormone extracted from a pituitary gland that had been deliberately contaminated with scrapie. However, because scrapie has such a long incubation period, the results would not be available for many months. In the meantime, the MRC weighed the theoretical risk of using growth hormone already purified from pituitaries that might be contaminated with CJD against the real risk of stopping the treatment for dwarfism. Thinking that the risk of CJD contamination was low, they decided to continue using growth hormone purified from pituitaries in the United Kingdom. Other countries were not even alerted of the risk.

The results of Dickinson's experiments turned out to be negative; mice showed no CJD infection. Nevertheless, cases of CJD did appear in humans who had been treated with growth hormone as children. The first case was reported in a California boy in 1984; two more cases soon followed. By a strange coincidence, this happened at about the same time that the first cases of BSE were surfacing among British cows.

By 1985, human growth hormone became available through the genetic engineering of bacteria, and the use of growth hormone extracted from pituitary glands stopped. However, the final tally in the number of CJD cases caused by contaminated growth hormone is not known. Because of the lengthy incubation period of CJD—in most cases, it takes about 12 years to incubate the disease, but an even longer time is possible—new cases of CJD among people who received pituitary growth hormone treatment as children are appearing every year. As of June 2003, the number stood at 161.

This tragedy prompted Brown, Gajdusek, and Gibbs to write an article, published in the *New England Journal of Medicine* in 1985, warning of the risks of passing CJD or other infectious diseases when transferring human tissue from one person to another. They were right to worry. In 1987, an American woman died of CJD, two years after receiving a supposedly contaminated dura mater (the outer membranes that cover the brain, which are used for patching after brain surgery). Six more cases were reported worldwide over the next five years. There had also been four cases of

CJD in women in Australia who had received gonadotropin, a hormone used to increase fertility.

The symptoms of CJD acquired iatrogenically are different from those of sporadic CJD. The earliest symptoms in the victims of iatrogenic CJD are problems with balance; this means that the cerebellum has been affected. On the other hand, sporadic CJD most often starts as dementia, which indicates that the frontal lobes of the brain are affected. Microscopic examination of the brain shows amyloid plaques in iatrogenic cases. These plaques are rarely seen in sporadic cases of CJD, but are common in kuru.

Both iatrogenic CJD and kuru involve peripheral infection; that is, the infection occurs by muscular injection (iatrogenic CJD) or orally (kuru), whereas sporadic CJD originates within the brain itself. Some scientists believe that peripheral infection could result in the selection of a particular strain of CJD that is different from the one that causes the sporadic form of the disease. It was not the first time that the existence of strains had been reported as an explanation for the appearance of different symptoms and pathologies in a TSE disease.

TSE STRAINS

Strains are slightly different versions of the same micro-organism (such as a virus or bacterium). Strains are the reason we need to get a flu shot every year, a vaccine specific to that year's dominant strain of the flu virus.

Several observations and experimental results suggest that there are also different strains within the TSE agents, each strain producing a characteristic set of symptoms in the infected human or animal, each with a specific incubation period. The existence of strains could be the reason why scrapie has received different names in different countries and at different times in history and why it took so long for scientists to recognize the different pathologies caused by CJD in humans as a single disease.

The possibility that the scrapie agent had different strains was suggested in the 1950s by Iain Pattison and Geoffrey C. Millson, two British veterinarians.[3] Pattison and Millson inoculated goats with brain tissue from scrapie-infected sheep. All the goats became infected, but they didn't all develop the same set of symptoms. The goats' symptoms fell into two groups: "drowsy" and "scratching." Drowsy goats had neurological symptoms from the onset, whereas scratching goats developed itching before the symptoms progressed to the neurological type.

Upon further experimentation, Pattison and Millson observed that goats inoculated with tissue from the brain of goats suffering from the scratching type of scrapie always developed scratching symptoms; goats inoculated with the drowsy type always developed neurological symptoms. These results seemed to suggest that there were two different strains of the scrapie agent.

Experiments with mice also support the idea that the scrapie agent has several strains. The existence of strains would agree with a fact that farmers have long known: that different breeds of sheep have varying degrees of susceptibility to scrapie.

As of 2003,[4] 20 TSE strains have been described experimentally, based on incubation time and the type of brain lesions they produce in rodents. In humans, as we have seen in Chapter 2, Gerstmann-Straüssler-Scheinker syndrome, fatal familial insomnia, and Creutzfeldt-Jakob disease produce different symptoms, incubation times, and pathological patterns in the brain, which suggests different strains may be involved.

With a conventional infectious agent, such as a bacterium or a virus (Figure 5.1), the different strains could be explained by **mutations**, accidental changes in the sequence of bases in their nucleic acid (see Chapter 6). But the TSE agent, researchers discovered, was anything but conventional. As we will see in Chapter 6, the TSE agent seemed not to have nucleic acid. If the TSE agent has no nucleic acid, how does it preserve

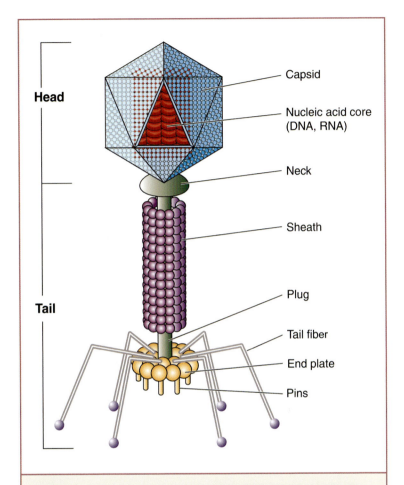

Head

Tail

Capsid

Nucleic acid core
(DNA, RNA)

Neck

Sheath

Plug

Tail fiber

End plate

Pins

Figure 5.1 Viruses are very small. More than 2,000 viruses like
the one in this diagram will fit into a single cell. Viruses are
parasites: They cannot multiply without first invading a host cell
and taking over its machinery to produce more virus particles.
Viruses infect every type of cell, from bacteria, algae, and fungi,
to protozoa, animals, and plants.

and transfer the information necessary to cause the different
symptoms and brain pathologies that scientists have observed?
Furthermore, if the TSE agent has no nucleic acid, then what is
it made of?

6

From Slow Virus to Prions

THE ELUSIVE AGENT

Infectious diseases are most often caused by parasites, fungi, bacteria, or viruses. By the mid-1960s, most scientists believed the TSE agent was a **virus** (a strand of nucleic acid inside a coat made of proteins. It was mainly a question of size; parasites, fungi, and bacteria are big enough to be seen with a microscope. Yet none could be seen in samples from TSE-infected tissue. Furthermore, Gajdusek and Gibbs, among other scientists, found infectivity in material that had been strained through a 0.22-micrometer pore filter. Viruses, whose size ranges from 0.02 to 0.25 micrometers, were the only ones small enough to pass through such filters.

If the TSE agent were a virus, then it was an unusual one: Viruses, like bacteria, are known to trigger an immune system reaction in infected individuals, but the TSE agent did not. Besides, most viruses can be seen with an electron microscope, but no virus had ever been seen in the brains of TSE victims.

Early attempts to purify the TSE agent failed. Separation techniques in the 1960s consisted of breaking the cells apart and separating their components into different fractions according to differences in their size, mass, weight, and solubility. But none of these methods worked for the TSE agent; it was present in all the parts. This made scientists wonder whether the TSE agent might be absorbed into the cell membranes. Because membranes are composed mainly of lipids (fatty matter), they tend to stick to everything during the purification process, which would explain why the agent was found everywhere.

CELLS AND VIRUSES

Animals and plants are made by cells—millions of cells of many different types. In contrast, most infectious agents are single-celled organisms and cannot be seen by the naked eye.

Cells are bounded by a membrane that separates them from the environment. The inside of a living cell is a thick, sticky fluid containing many tiny structures whose perfectly coordinated activity keeps the cell alive. In cells called eukaryotes (Figure 6.1b), one of these structures, the nucleus, has several (from four to hundreds) linear strands of a long sequence of deoxyribonucleic acid (DNA)—the genetic material that passes traits from one generation to the next. Each strand is tightly packed to form a **chromosome**.

Not all cells have a nucleus. Those that don't, such as bacteria, are called prokaryotes (Figure 6.1a). In a prokaryotic cell, the genetic material consists of a unique circular strand of DNA.

Unlike bacteria or other parasites, viruses are not cells. They are large particles made up of many equal subunits. Viruses have two components: an external shell (capsid) made of proteins and a core that consists of one or more nucleic acid strands of either DNA or ribonucleic acid (RNA), another form of genetic material.

Viruses cannot reproduce by themselves or perform any other vital functions. They remain unchanged until they come into contact with a cell that they can use as a host. They then attach themselves to its surface and inject their nucleic acid inside. The viral nucleic acid directs the cell to make more viral nucleic acid and new capsid proteins. Eventually, new virus particles are assembled and released into the body of the host organism, such as an animal or human.

Proteins on the viral capsids stimulate the immune system of the host cell to produce antibodies. Antibodies can neutralize the virus and protect the organism against future infections by the same type of virus. Antibodies in the blood are also used in various diagnostic tests to identify which microorganism is causing a particular infectious disease.

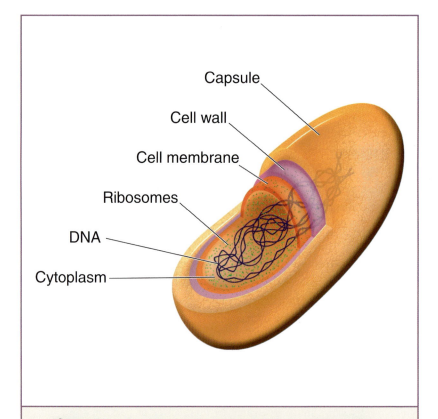

Figure 6.1a Compared to the eukaryotic cells, prokaryotic cells are small. They basically consist of a cell envelope (very different chemically from eukaryotic cell walls), a protoplasm that contains ribosomes and a nucleoid, and often have projections called pili or flagella. Although they lack the nucleus and other organelles present in eukaryotic cells, prokaryotic cells are complex microorganisms. The fact that they have survived on Earth for 3.5 billion years indicates the extraordinary adaptability of their cellular structure and function.

The agent was unusual in other ways, too. As Gajdusek pointed out in his Nobel Prize acceptance speech in 1976, the TSE pathogen was incredibly resistant. This resistance had caused the unwanted contamination with scrapie of 1,500 of the 18,000 sheep that had received the loup vaccine made

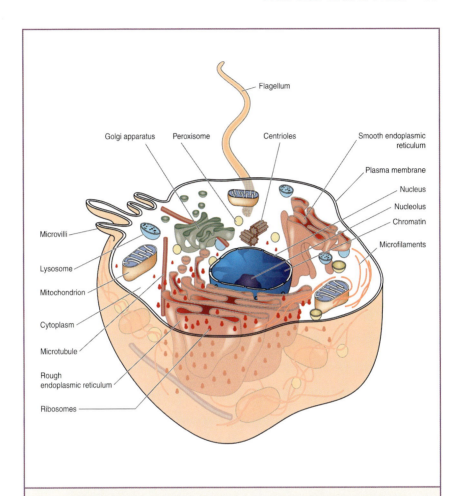

Figure 6.1b A eukaryote cell (seen here) is a complex, compartmentalized unit that contains a nucleus and other specialized structures called organelles. Bacteria and viruses are much simpler organisms. Bacteria are prokaryotes, meaning they have no nucleus. Viruses are even less complex—they are not even considered cells, just particles of genetic matter.

in 1935 and 1936 (see Chapter 4). The sheep brain used to prepare the vaccine had been treated with formaldehyde, a chemical that destroys all microorganisms, including viruses. Yet, it had failed to kill the scrapie agent.

The TSE agent was not destroyed by freezing or by boiling (100° C [212° F] for 30 minutes) the samples that contained it, nor by dry-heating the samples at 600° C (1,112° F). The same team exposed scrapie-infected brain tissue in water to ultraviolet (UV) light (254 nanometers). UV light of this wavelength causes nucleic acids to break apart. Yet it had no effect on the infectivity of the TSE samples.

More impressive still: Blasting scrapie-infected tissue with high-energy beams of electrons (an elemental particle with a negative electrical charge) didn't destroy its infectivity either. Such electron beams have enough energy to knock electrons from the atoms in the sample and transform the atoms into positive and negative ions; that is why this technique is called **ionizing radiation**. Ionizing radiation is used to calculate the size of an infectious agent. The smaller the agent, the higher the radiation dose necessary to inactivate it. Researchers found that "the agent was smaller, perhaps by a factor of 10, than any known virus."[1]

During the 1960s, researchers also demonstrated that exposing samples of scrapie brain with enzymes known to damage nucleic acids produced no reduction in infectivity. However, exposing the samples to enzymes known to damage proteins reduced infectivity dramatically—by more that 90%. Was it possible that the scrapie agent was an infectious protein? An infectious protein with no nucleic acid?[2] Nucleic acids are needed for replication (making copies of a cell or virus). And the scrapie agent was obviously making more copies of itself in the infected human or animal.

Besides, the fact that there seemed to be different strains both in scrapie and in human CJD implied that nucleic acid was present. Proteins do not have a known mechanism by which to encode the information needed to produce different strains. Only nucleic acids do. At least, that is what the central dogma of molecular biology tells us. Before we can argue this point further, however, we need some background information to understand why scientists believed so strongly that this is so.

THE GENETIC CODE

For a species to survive, its individuals must reproduce—that is, make others similar to themselves that will survive and continue to reproduce after they die. Because, among thousands of other reasons, children tend to look like their parents, and seeds from an apple always grow into apple trees, it was obvious that something was passed from the progenitor (parent or tree) to its offspring that carried the information to make one of its own. What this something was no one knew.

In the 19th century, while experimenting with peas, Austrian botanist Gregor Mendel realized that the traits he was studying (green or yellow color, rough or smooth surface) were passed on as independent entities to the progeny (offspring). He named these theoretical entities that carried the information "genes." What these genes were or how they carried the information remained unknown.

By the middle of the 20th century, it had already been established that these genes were stored in the cell nucleus in individual units called chromosomes, and that these chromosomes were made of proteins and an acid called deoxyribonucleic acid (DNA). Of the two, DNA was more abundant. But DNA, made in fixed proportions of sugar, phosphate, and four different bases, didn't seem to have enough variability to store information. Proteins, on the other hand, are complex molecules. They consist of chains made out of 20 basic units called **amino acids**. Twenty amino acids, scientists thought, could provide enough variability to make up a code and carry information. Because of this, proteins were believed to be the genetic carriers.

So strong was this belief, that when, in the late 1920s, Frederick Griffith ran an experiment (Figure 6.2) that showed that a strain of nucleic acid from a dead virulent (powerful)

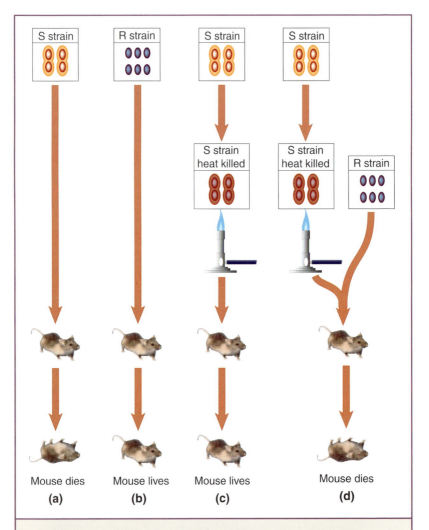

Figure 6.2 Griffith experimented with the bacterium *Streptococcus pneumoniae*, which has two strains: with a capsule, or smooth (S); and without a capsule, or rough (R). Only the S strain is virulent; mice infected with the S strain die. When the S strain is heated, it loses its virulence. Griffith showed that when the nonvirulent R strain and the preheated S strain are coinoculated, the mice die. Why? Because, once in the mouse's body, the R strain has acquired DNA from the S strain, the part that codes for the capsule and, as a result, has become virulent.

strain of bacteria could transform a nonvirulent bacteria strain into a virulent one, his experiment was ignored.

This apparent contradiction was brilliantly solved in 1953 by James Watson and Francis Crick, two young scientists working at Cambridge University, England. Their conclusions, published in a one-page paper in *Nature*,[3] opened a new field in biology, the field of molecular biology.

In his controversial book, *The Double Helix*, Watson recounts the reasoning and sometimes unconventional methods of work that led him and Crick to their famous model of DNA (Figure 6.3).[4] Watson was convinced that the DNA in a chromosome consisted of two strands of DNA. (After all, reproduction usually requires two parents, and chromosomes in the cell also come in pairs). After countless discussions, and the building of several models for the DNA structure, Watson and Crick came to the conclusion that the only way to explain all the data available was that the DNA structure must be made out of two chains twisted around each other in the form of a double helix (spiral pattern).

In this double helix, the sides of the "ladder" are made of alternating molecules of sugar and phosphate, each rung formed by two of the four nitrogenous bases available—adenine (A), guanine (G), thymine (T), and cytosine (C)—facing each other. The two bases that form the rungs are held together by weak hydrogen bonds (Figure 6.4).

The mysterious genetic code, the language used by cells to pass information to the next generation, had been unraveled. According to Watson and Crick's model, the genetic code was stored as a long sequence of bases in a strand of DNA. A typical sequence might be something like ATTAGCCAGTCAATGGGCCCAAAATTT.

DNA MAKES RNA; RNA MAKES PROTEIN

Watson and Crick also realized that the bases could bind to each other in only two combinations: T to A and G to C. This

(continued on page 70)

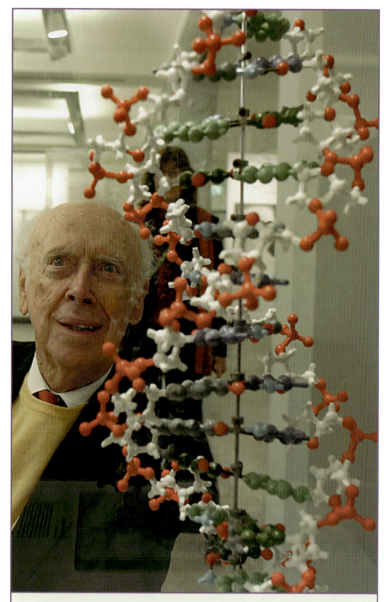

Figure 6.3 James Watson is shown here with a model of the DNA structure, on October 11, 2004. In 1953, Watson, along with his research partner Francis Crick, discovered the double helix structure of DNA.

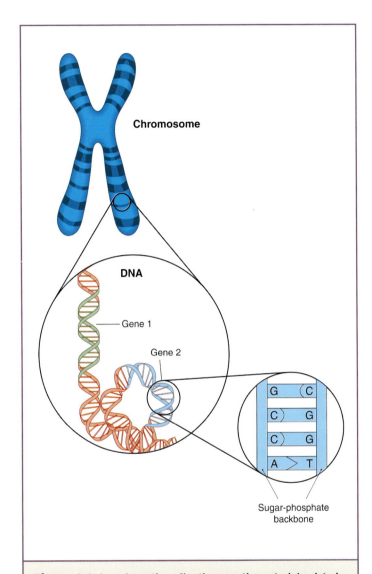

Figure 6.4 In eukaryotic cells, the genetic material exists in several linear molecules of deoxyribonucleic acid (DNA). These linear DNA molecules are associated with proteins that form the chromosomes. A DNA molecule is made of nucleotides. Each nucleotide contains a sugar, a phosphate, and one of four nitrogen bases. Each DNA molecule contains many different genes.

(continued from page 67)

meant that the sequence of bases in any given strand had to be complementary to the sequence in the opposite strand.

It did not escape the researchers that this restriction in the base-paring combination provided a way for the DNA to replicate (make copies of) itself. Upon separation of both strands, each DNA strand would be able to form a complementary copy of itself by binding to free nucleotide bases. (**Nucleotides** are defined as the individual units that make up DNA. Each nucleotide has a sugar, a phosphate, and a nitrogenous base.) So the question to be answered was this: How did this long sequence of only four nucleotides contain the information for the thousands of proteins that make up a living organism? If we consider that every protein, however long or complicated it may seem, is made out of 20 amino acids, the question can be rephrased as: How can 4 "letters" (4 nucleotides) specify 20 amino acids? In pure mathematical terms, the simplest answer was: Three letters code for an amino acid. Why? Because, there are 20 amino acids and 4 letters. If every letter were to code for one specific amino acid, the combinations could only make four amino acids (one amino acid for each of the four letters); if two letters were needed, they would make 16 ($4 \times 4 = 16$). With three letters, there are 64 possibilities ($4 \times 4 \times 4 = 64$). 64 is a bigger number than the 20 amino acids that exist. That could be explained if more than a triplet of nucleotides would code for the same amino acid. Data soon confirmed that, in fact, every amino acid is determined by a sequence of three nucleotides.

Later experiments also provided information on how the synthesis of a protein really happens in the cell: The process is twofold. First, the long strand of DNA is copied into shorter, single-stranded chains of different nucleic acids called mRNA (messenger ribonucleic acid); each chain of mRNA is the model for a specific protein. The translation of the mRNA into proteins is a complex process that requires protein-assembly machines known as ribosomes and another strand of RNA called **tRNA**. Different tRNA molecules carry the amino acids one at a time to the ribosomes in the order specified by the sequence of nucleotides that makes up the mRNA. Therefore, it was established that the genetic information to make proteins is carried in the sequence of bases in the DNA and that the transfer of information is a one-way street, from DNA to protein (Figure 6.5). As Francis Crick put it: "DNA makes RNA; RNA makes protein." According to this principle, protein never makes protein, protein never makes RNA, and protein never makes DNA.

Yet Crick knew there was something in nature that even this model could not explain: "There is, for example," Crick wrote, "the problem of the chemical nature of the agent of the disease scrapie . . . "[5] There seemed to be an agent, seemingly a protein, that was able to replicate itself without nucleic acid.

PRIONS

The 1970s were a period of frustration for those studying the TSE agent. All attempts to isolate the agent failed, and its nature remained a mystery. In 1972, Stanley B. Prusiner, a graduate chemist studying neurology at the University of California at San Francisco, School of Medicine, encountered TSE for the first time in one of his patients who was suffering from CJD. Fascinated by the mysterious disease, Prusiner set out to learn all he could about it. "The amazing properties of the presumed causative 'slow virus,'" he would later write, "captivated my imagination and I began to think that defining the molecular structure of this elusive agent might be a wonderful research project."[6]

Prusiner started a collaboration with scrapie experts William Hadlow and Carl M. Eklund, both from the National Institutes of Health's Rocky Mountain Laboratories. Their first attempts at purifying the agent from infected mice brains

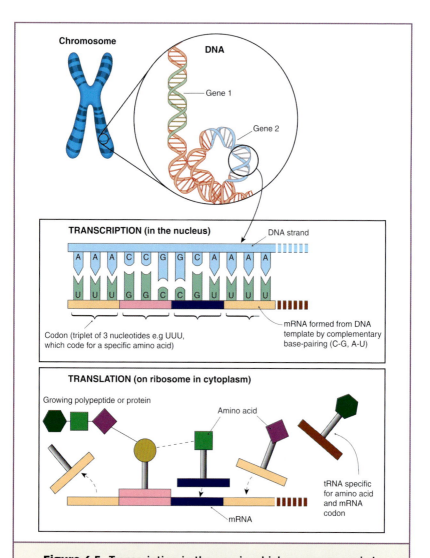

Figure 6.5 Transcription is the way in which genes are copied into RNA. During transcription, individual nucleotides that are complementary to the ones in the DNA link are sequentially converted into a chain. During translation, amino acids are brought to the mRNA molecule by a transfer RNA (tRNA). The tRNA binds to the mRNA molecule at one end; at the other, it carries a specific amino acid. After its amino acid has joined the growing protein chain, the tRNA moves away.

met the same difficulties that their predecessors had encountered. The scrapie agent seemed to be in all the fractions, and the long incubation period of the disease made the research impossibly slow. But in 1978, Prusiner and his colleagues introduced two changes. First, they switched the experimental animal from mice to hamsters. Because hamsters develop the disease in half the time that mice do, this change shortened the research time. Second, instead of diluting the infectious sample up to 10 times and inoculating every dilution into 6 different animals as other researchers were doing, Prusiner's team inoculated 4 animals with a sample whose concentration they had previously determined. This meant that "instead of observing 60 animals for a year, we could assay a sample with just four animals in 60 days."[7] Thanks to these improvements, Prusiner and his colleagues performed more experiments with the scrapie agent than anyone had ever done in the previous 200 years.

In 1981, Prusiner and his team obtained a purified preparation that was 5,000 to 10,000 times more effective in producing the disease than the initial cellular extract was. Consistent with previous findings, the infectivity of the sample was not affected by chemicals that destroy or modify nucleic acids, such as nucleases, zinc ions, and hydroxylamine. But it was destroyed by those that affect proteins.

Up to 95% of this purified fraction corresponded to a specific protein. If this protein was indeed the scrapie agent, as Prusiner's team believed, the agent would be 100 times smaller than any known virus.

In his search to learn about TSEs, Prusiner visited Gajdusek in Papua New Guinea in 1978 and in 1981. By his second visit, both Gajdusek and Prusiner had reached the conclusion that the TSE agent was a protein. But they lacked definitive proof, since they could not totally rule out whether some nucleic acid was still present in the purified preparations protected by the protein.

Gajdusek thought it would be premature to give the agent a name until they were certain of its nature. But Prusiner decided not to wait. Back in the United States, Prusiner published his results in the April 9, 1982, issue of *Science*, and named this new infectious agent a **prion**. He chose the name *prion* (pronounced pree-on) for "proteinaceous infectious particles" to emphasize his belief that the agent was a protein. He also mentioned in the article the

FROM SEQUENCE OF AMINO ACIDS TO ACTIVE PROTEIN

A protein emerges from the translation process as a long chain of amino acids. The sequence of amino acids that makes up this chain is called the primary structure of the protein (Figure 6.6). It is this sequence that determines the biological function of the protein molecule: what the protein does. A change in only one amino acid in the sequence can alter or destroy the activity of the protein.

After it is made, the protein folds into a secondary structure as hydrogen bonds form between every fourth amino acid in the chain. The specific sequence of amino acids in each protein determines which parts of the protein will fold as a right-handed coil structure (an alpha-helix), which will take the shape of pleated sheets (beta sheets), and which will remain unstructured.

Some proteins can be described by their primary and secondary structures. Others are more complex. By a process not yet totally understood, these proteins fold themselves into a three-dimensional structure (tertiary structure), which is determined somewhat, but not totally, by the sequence of amino acids.

In some cases, several proteins join together to form dimers, trimers, or polymers in what is called the quaternary structure.

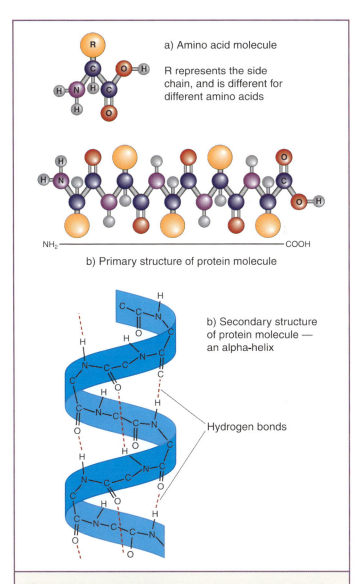

a) Amino acid molecule

R represents the side chain, and is different for different amino acids

NH₂ ———————————— COOH

b) Primary structure of protein molecule

b) Secondary structure of protein molecule — an alpha-helix

Hydrogen bonds

Figure 6.6 Proteins are long sequences of amino acids. The sequence of amino acids constitutes the primary structure of the protein. As shown in the figure above, segments of the protein can fold into different shapes, forming alpha-helix, beta sheets, or random coils. This is what is called the secondary structure.

possibility that a small nucleic acid could still be present within a shell of protein.

"Prions," he wrote, "are small proteinaceous infectious particles which are resistant to inactivation by most procedures that modify nucleic acids. The term 'prion' underscores the requirement of a protein for infection; current knowledge does not allow exclusion of a small nucleic acid within the interior of the particle."[8]

Fifteen years later, in 1997, Prusiner would receive the Nobel Prize for his work. But when his paper first appeared, it was met with skepticism and resistance by the scientific community. British researchers were particularly upset. They felt Prusiner's work had not contributed new evidence toward identifying the TSE agent. They also believed that to give it a name that reinforced the idea that it was a protein would cloud the objectivity in the search for the nature of the agent.

Alan Dickinson at the MRC Neuropathogenesis Unit in Edinburgh was particularly outraged. He criticized Prusiner's conclusions in a *Lancet* editorial. Among other points, Dickinson reminded Prusiner that the protein-only hypothesis for the TSE agent did not explain the existence of strains—its ability to produce different incubation times and patterns of brain lesions in its victims.

In the early 1980s[9], Dickinson, George W. Outram, and Richard Kimberlin proposed an alternative theory on the nature of the TSE agent. According to their theory, the TSE agent was a **virino**, a very small virus without a protein coat. Some plant viruses, called **viroids**, do exist. They are only bits of RNA. But even though viroids are about one-tenth the size of the smallest virus known to date, they are too big to comply with the properties of the TSE agent. The virino would have to be even smaller, Dickinson and his colleagues theorized, just a bit of nucleic acid that does not code for its own protein, but takes it instead from the host cell. In this way, the virino would not be recognized as a foreign particle by the host and thus escape the body's defenses.

As of the early 2000s, the virino has yet to be identified. The possibility that a strand of nucleic acid exists within the prion has not been ruled out either.

7

More on Prions

PRION AGGREGATES AND AMYLOID PLAQUES

During the process of **purifying** (separating the agent from other components) the scrapie agent, Prusiner's team had been puzzled by the fact that the infectious particles seemed to be both smaller than any known virus and bigger than a bacterium (see relative sizes of bacteria and viruses in Figure 7.1). The explanation for this became clear when they realized that the prion proteins could bind together and form rod-shaped particles of up to 1,000 molecules.

Taking this finding one step further, they speculated that accumulations of these rod-shaped particles might form the amyloid plaques often found in the brains of TSE victims (see Chapter 3). In Prusiner's own words: "The amyloid plaques observed in transmissible degenerative neurological diseases might consist of prions." [1]

Prusiner and his colleagues were not the first to discover these particles or to make the connection between them and the amyloid plaques in the brain. Patricia Merz, working in collaboration with Robert Somerville in Edinburgh, had seen similar structures under the electron microscope back in 1978. These tiny, stick-like filaments or fibrils seemed to be made by even thinner filaments. Always present in samples from scrapie-infected mice brains, but never in those from healthy animals, the fibril concentration increased as the disease progressed.

Merz named these aggregates "scrapie-associated fibrils," or SAF (Figure 7.2). [2] Not knowing what they were made of, and because, although they were only visible under the electron microscope, they had a similar structure to the much bigger amyloid plaques (amyloid

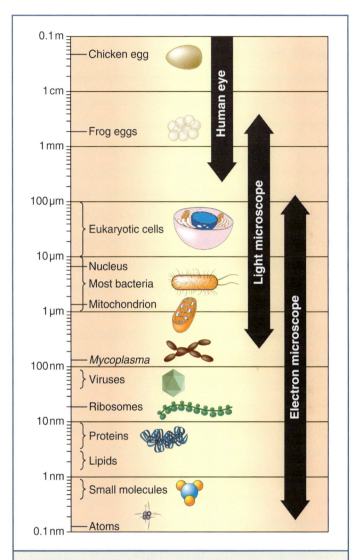

0.1 m — Chicken egg

1 cm — Frog eggs

1 mm

100 μm — Eukaryotic cells

10 μm — Nucleus
       — Most bacteria
       — Mitochondrion
1 μm

100 nm — *Mycoplasma*
       } Viruses
       — Ribosomes
10 nm — } Proteins
       } Lipids
1 nm — } Small molecules

0.1 nm — Atoms

Human eye

Light microscope

Electron microscope

Figure 7.1 As illustrated in the figure above, bacteria are visible under a light microscope, while viruses require the use of a high-powered electron microscope. The scrapie agent puzzled scientists because sometimes it seemed to be bigger than bacteria, and at other times, seemed smaller than a virus. This strange trait was explained when researchers realized the agent was a protein that could accumulate in great numbers.

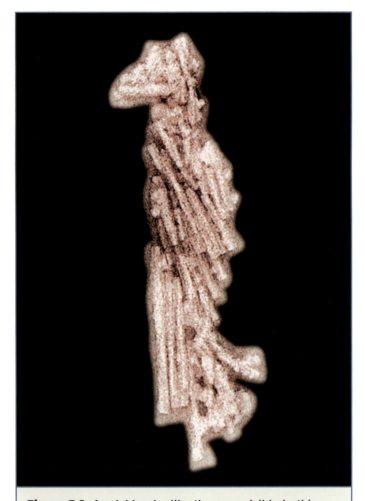

Figure 7.2 Amyloid rods, like the ones visible in this image seen through an electron microscope, are present in tissue preparations from the brains of CJD patients and of cows infected with BSE. Amyloid rods are made by up to 1,000 prion molecules.

plaques are visible under a less powerful light microscope), she speculated that the SAF could also be made of amyloid.

When stained with Congo red dye, amyloid glows green under polarized light. Merz's SAF did not. But that didn't deter Merz from believing that the fibrils were made of amyloid. She blamed the failure of this test on the small size and low concentration of the fibrils in the scrapie samples. Later experiments would prove she was right.

Working with a more purified preparation, Prusiner succeeded in staining the rods with Congo red. He also managed to produce antibodies against the prion protein by injecting a highly concentrated sample in rabbits. Once purified, the antibodies were found to bind specifically to the amyloid rods. This could only mean that Prusiner's rods were indeed made of prions. Although Prusiner denied that SAF and amyloid rods are the same, Merz proved otherwise by showing that both structures react identically to the prion antibodies.[3]

In 1987, SAF were also found in brain samples from cows infected with BSE by scientists working for MAFF Central Veterinary Laboratory in Surrey, near London.

CELLULAR PRION/INFECTIOUS PRION

During the second half of the 1980s, Prusiner continued to study the prion, the protein he believed to be the TSE agent. Working with Leroy E. Hood of the California Institute of Technology and Charles Weissmann of the University of Zurich, Prusiner determined the prion's amino acid sequence. The prion protein consisted of 253 amino acids, a number close to the 300 the researchers had previously estimated based on its molecular weight.

As explained in Chapter 6, each amino acid is encoded in the genome (the full set of genes) by a sequence of three nucleotides. This means that once the sequence of amino acids of any protein is known, it is possible to determine the sequence of nucleotides of the gene that codes for it.

Using the then-new techniques of molecular biology, Prusiner, Hood, and Weissmann designed an experiment to test whether the prion gene was present in the cellular genome of infected animals.

The experiment met with success. Prusiner and his colleagues soon found that the gene for the prion protein was, indeed, present in the genome of scrapie-infected hamsters. But, to their surprise, they also found the same gene in healthy hamsters.[4] At about the same time, other researchers also detected the prion gene in the brain cells of healthy mice[5] and humans.

How could this be possible? How could the gene coding for the prion protein be present in healthy animals? And if it was, why didn't those animals develop the disease as well? Maybe, researchers thought, the prion gene was not being expressed (it didn't make protein) in healthy animals. This was not the case, though. After further experiments, they realized that the gene was being actively transcribed into mRNA in healthy animals, and, using antibodies against the prion protein, they found the prion protein in the brains of both sick and healthy animals. But the protein from healthy animals did not behave in the same way as the prion in animals that showed symptoms of a TSE.

First, in healthy animals, the prion protein was present in lower quantities. Second, the prion protein from healthy animals was destroyed by proteinase K (see explanation below), whereas the prion protein from TSE-infected animals was only partially digested by it. After treatment with the protease, the protein got smaller, but there was still a core of 27,000 to 30,000 daltons (one dalton is the weight of a hydrogen atom, or about 1.66×10^{-24} gram), which seemed to be resistant to further digestion.

Proteases are enzymes that specifically digest proteins by breaking the bonds between amino acids. Proteinase K is a protease. A difference in the susceptibility to digestion by proteinase K of two proteins with the same sequence of amino acids could be explained only if they had a different configuration—a different shape—in which the amino acid bonds could not be digested because they were not accessible to the protease.

The idea of having two different configurations for a single sequence of amino acids was disregarded at the time. According to the principles of molecular biology, the sequence of amino acids determines the way the protein folds into its secondary and tertiary structure. Still, a difference in configuration seemed to be the only explanation to fit these data.

In 1993, Fred Cohen, together with Prusiner and other colleagues at the University of California at San Francisco, showed that the cellular prion protein (PrP^C) and the lethal version (or PrP^{Sc}) do have different configurations. The term *PrP^{Sc}* was chosen to name scrapie prion protein, although it now refers to any pathological prion. The normal prion consists mainly of alpha helices and a few or no beta sheets, while the lethal prion consists mainly of beta sheets (see box on page 74 and Figure 6.6).

In 1996 and 1997, Rudolf Glockshuber, Kurt Wuthrich, and their groups in Zurich[6] crystallized prion proteins and observed the prion's true structure. The protein is folded into three alpha helices and two small beta sheets (refer again to the box on page 74), whereas the first half of the chain— about 100 amino acids long—remains unstructured. The conformation of the infectious prion protein has not yet been determined.

MUTATIONS ON THE PRION PROTEIN AND THEIR EFFECT ON TSE

Circumstantial evidence indicating that the prion protein was the agent responsible for causing TSE continued to accumulate during the second half of the 1980s. However, the definitive proof that the prion was the only cause of TSE would be to synthesize (create) the protein *in vitro* (outside a living body, in a laboratory setting) and then to reproduce the disease by inoculating this synthetic protein.

The Prusiner group was eager to try this approach. But the experiment turned out to be more difficult than the researchers had anticipated. By 1986, Prusiner wrote:

> . . . we knew the plan would not work. For one thing, it proved very difficult to induce the gene to make the high levels of PrP needed for conducting studies. For another thing, the protein that was produced was the normal, cellular form—PrP^C—rather than the infectious, "scrapie" form PrP^{Sc}. Fortunately work on a different problem led us to an alternative approach.[7]

The problem Prusiner was referring to was the existence of hereditary types of human CJD: Gerstmann-Straüssler-Scheinker syndrome (GSS), fatal familial insomnia, and familial CJD. In 1988, Karen Hsiao, one of Prusiner's graduate students, determined the sequence of nucleotides of the prion gene from a brain sample of a man suffering from GSS. The gene differed from the normal prion in just one nucleotide. This same point mutation (difference in a single nucleotide) was also found in several other GSS patients. The mutation, a change in the 102nd codon, causes the normal protein leucine (L) to be replaced by the amino acid proline (P). "We established," Prusiner wrote, "genetic linkage between the mutation and the disease finding that strongly implies the mutation is the cause."[8]

To prove this point further, Hsiao created a line of mice whose prion genes had been cut and replaced with the human GSS prion. These mice that had the mutated prion protein of the GSS gene spontaneously developed a spongiform disease.

Apparently, a single-point mutation in the protein had transformed the cellular prion protein into a lethal form. This probably happened, researchers speculated, because the mutation caused the protein to fold into a shape that the cellular proteases could not degrade.

By the late 1990s, scientists had discovered 13 different point mutations and 9 other types of mutations (i.e., mutations that produce a shorter or longer protein) on the cellular prion protein that also resulted in the onset of CJD in humans.

The different mutations in the prion protein (Figure 7.3) correlated with differences in the clinical course and neuropathology of the disease. For example, different mutations meant differences in the age at which the victim will get the disease and the length of time (from months to decades) it would take the disease to kill its victim. These mutations also determined the type of symptoms—whether the patient would develop dementia, muscle incoordination and slurring, or insomnia—and the number of holes and the presence or absence of amyloid plaques in the brain.

Point mutations that affect the onset and type of disease have also been found in animals. In mice, some mutations determine the incubation period and the site of lesions within the brain; in sheep, they determine the incubation period and the susceptibility to infection.

Differences in the sequence of amino acids have also been found between hamsters and mice prions. Some researchers suggest that these differences could be responsible for the species barrier that exists in animals against prions from another species.

HOW DOES THE INFECTIOUS PRION PROTEIN MAKE MORE OF ITS OWN?

The role of the cellular prion protein is not known. The fact that it has been found in the brain cells of all animals tested (not only mammals such as sheep, mice, hamsters, and humans, but also chickens and turtles) suggests that it must perform some essential function. Yet, mice that lack the genes for the prion protein and, as a consequence, do not produce the cellular prion protein, are healthy and don't seem to be any different from normal mice. There is one exception: Mice created in the laboratory without the prion protein do not develop scrapie after being inoculated with an infectious sample. This result implies that the cellular prion protein is necessary for the TSE infection to proceed. Scientists believe that this is because prions do not reproduce inside the cells the way other infectious agents, such as viruses and bacteria, do. They do not form new copies of themselves; instead, they convert the cellular proteins into their own configuration, a configuration that is resistant to being broken down by cellular proteases.

When mice that lack only one of the copies of the prion protein gene (every cell has two sets of chromosomes; there-fore, there are two copies of every gene) are inoculated with scrapie prion protein, they develop scrapie, but the incubation time of the disease is longer. This is to be expected if we consider that cells with only one copy of the gene would take longer to make the same amount of protein than cells with two copies would. Therefore, the infectious prion would have less protein to transform and the infection would proceed at a slower rate.

The first step in the conversion of the cellular prion into an infectious one requires that the two proteins bind together. The exact way in which the proteins bind and how the con-version proceeds are not known.

According to one theory—the template-direct model proposed by Prusiner—the cellular prion may exist in the cell in an intermediate, unstructured state. This intermediate form interacts first with another protein—protein X, and this union allows the intermediate cellular prion to bind to the infectious prion. Then, the intermediate cellular prion adopts the configuration of the infectious prion and becomes infectious itself.

Several findings support this theory. For instance, for years, researchers had tried to transform cellular prion into

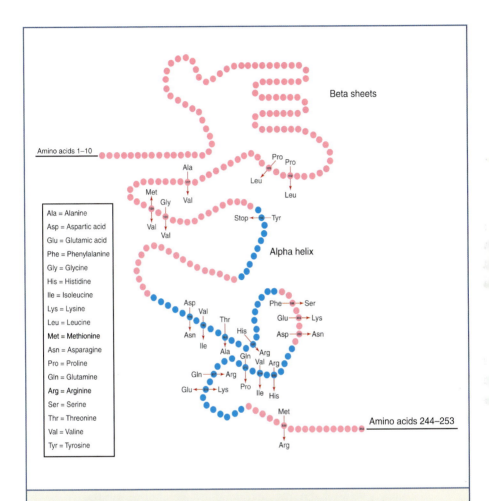

Figure 7.3 This figure shows the 253 amino acids of the human prion protein, illustrating which regions of the protein form pleated sheets (beta sheet configuration) and which are folded into a right-handed coil structure (alpha helix configuration). The location of some of the point mutation found in pathogenic prion proteins (and the amino acid changes they cause) are also seen here.

the pathogenic prion in the test tube by mixing the two proteins together. The experiments were unsuccessful until they had the idea of destroying the configuration of the proteins before adding the infectious prion to the mixture. After they did this, the cellular prion took on the configuration of the pathogenic prion.

Even before Prusiner had coined the term *prion* for the TSE agent in the 1982 article, Gajdusek had proposed a model to explain the way TSE diseases progress. In his theory—the nucleate polymerization model—Gajdusek compared the propagation of the CJD agent to crystal formation. He proposed that the invading TSE agent was like a crystal and that the cellular protein adhered to this crystal, and consequently adopted its conformation. As new units joined the crystal, it continued to grow until it formed the scrapie-associated fibrils that Merz detected in scrapie-infected brain samples under the electron microscope. According to his theory, the crystal did not grow forever, and eventually, either because of the intervention of an external agent or because the structure itself had become unstable, the crystal broke into smaller pieces. Each of these pieces would later serve as a seed to recruit other cellular prion proteins.

In the nucleate polymerization model, even the appearance of strains without a nucleic acid poses no problem. Charles Weissmann explains: "The seeding hypothesis says that the infectious agent is really an assembly of molecules— simply a crystal. So the idea is that, depending on the structure of the crystal the molecules that add to it will adapt to whatever the conformation is."[9] As of today, Gajdusek's polymerization theory is the one most widely accepted.

THE TSE AGENT: PRION OR VIRINO?

The prion-only theory gained support steadily over the years as experiments in different laboratories accumulated data that supported it. This theory could explain, for instance, the puzzling fact that the TSE diseases do not elicit an immune response. If the prion protein exists naturally in the cells, the

KISS OF DEATH OR ICE NINE?

Prions are not the only proteins capable of causing disease. The toxins produced by the bacteria that cause diphtheria, anthrax, and botulism are also proteins, and they can kill.

The difference between prions and toxins is that the amount of toxin remains the same throughout the course of the illness, whereas prions multiply and accumulate as the disease progresses. It is this ability to multiply, apparently without the need for nucleic acid, which made the prion theory hard to accept back in 1982.

Since then, two theories have been proposed that accommodate both the molecular biology postulate—"DNA makes RNA; RNA makes protein"—and the fact that prion proteins do multiply in the victim's body. Both theories propose that prions do not really make new molecules, but instead convert their cellular counterparts to their own lethal conformation.

For Prusiner, this conversion takes place in a one-to-one interaction between a cellular protein and a lethal prion. In this interaction, which some researchers have named the "Kiss of Death," the proteins bind, and "kiss"; this kiss changes the conformation of the normal prion into the conformation of the lethal one. Then, the two prion molecules separate and each goes on to bind another cellular prion, and the process is repeated.

For Gajdusek, the lethal prion is the seed of a crystal. Cellular prions bind to this seed and adopt its shape as the crystal grows. This process, Gadjusek believes, is not unlike the formation of "Ice Nine," the unmeltable ice Kurt Vonnegut[*] describes in his novel *Cat's Cradle*. "Ice Nine" is a form of ice with a melting point so high that, once water has crystallized into this conformation, it will remain frozen forever, unable to sustain life.

[*] Vonnegut, Kurt. *Cat's Cradle*, originally published in 1963.

body would not react against the invading prion because it would recognize it as one of its own proteins. Mice that lack the gene for the prion protein do produce antibodies when inoculated with the prion protein and develop an immune response of sorts with inflammation and fever.

It can also explain the seemingly contradictory findings that TSE diseases are both hereditary and infectious. The disease is hereditary when a mutation in the gene of the cellular prion protein produces a protein with a slightly different sequence of amino acids—a protein that on its own may fold into an infectious shape. The disease is infectious when a foreign prion enters the body and changes the cellular protein to its lethal shape.

As for the existence of strains of TSE—the main flaw in the prion theory, according to Dickinson and other scientists back in 1982—it doesn't bother Prusiner at all. A prion, he argues, could fold itself in different conformations, each producing different symptoms and brain lesions.

Still, the definitive proof that the prion is the only agent of the TSE disease is still lacking. Several experiments performed in the 1990s, in which PrP^{Sc} obtained in vitro was inoculated into mice, failed to produce infection. This failure prompted Charles Weissmann to conclude that, "PrP [prion protein] is essential but not sufficient,"[10] and Prusiner to suggest that a cofactor, a "chaperone molecule" which he calls "protein X," is necessary to help cellular prion protein fold into the PrP^{Sc} conformation. To date, protein X has not been found.

There are other researchers who, like Robert G. Rohwer at the Veterans' Affairs Maryland Health Care System in Baltimore, still refuse to believe that the prion protein is the TSE agent. The theory will not be proven until, Rohwer says, someone "can create infectivity de novo in the test tube." But if the proponents of the prion theory have failed to find the ultimate proof that the prion alone is sufficient to cause

TSE, the proponents of the virino theory as the TSE agent have not succeeded either in producing a piece of nucleic acid that would cause the disease. And so, even though the prion theory is widely accepted today, the debate on the nature of the TSE agent is still open.

8

Mad Cow Disease Revisited

BSE: ONE AMONG MANY

Despite the gaps that still exist in the field of TSE research, a great deal more is known today about these diseases than was known two decades ago.

We know, for instance, why the cows started to act strangely that winter of 1984–1985. It was because the neurons in their cerebellum (the part of the brain that controls balance and movement) and other regions of their brain were dying. We know the neurons were dying because a prion, a pathological protein, was turning their normal cellular prions to its own lethal conformation—a conformation the cellular proteases could not destroy.

We know all this because, for centuries, veterinarians in Europe had been studying scrapie, a strange disease that affects sheep, and because doctors in Germany in the 1920s had found a human neuronal degenerative disease that they had named CJD. Further evidence surfaced in the 1950s, when members of the Fore, a Stone Age tribe in Papua New Guinea that practiced cannibalism, started to die of a disease they called kuru, which means "trembling with fear."

All these diseases were found to be related to the bovine spongiform encephalopathy (BSE) that in the 1980s turned the cows mad in the United Kingdom. It was because researchers had already been studying these diseases that the link between BSE and vCJD (the name BSE receives when it affects humans) was promptly detected and was the reason that further spread of BSE among cows and vCJD among humans was averted.

Most researchers now believe that all TSE diseases are caused by prions. A prion is a protein that can exist in two conformations: a normal one that is present in healthy cells and a lethal one that causes disease.

In some cases, the pathological prion has the same amino acid sequence as the cellular one. This is the case with kuru and sporadic CJD. In other cases, the prion proteins differ. For instance, the victims of the familial forms of CJD, Gerstmann-Straüssler-Scheinker syndrome, and fatal familial insomnia have point mutations in their prion genes which translate into one amino acid difference in the sequence of amino acids of the prion protein. According to Gajdusek, this single amino acid difference lowers the chances for the spontaneous folding of the normal protein into a pathological conformation.

Mutations have also been found among animal prions. Sometimes the mutation is just a point mutation in the gene— that is, a single amino acid change in the prion protein; at other times, the lethal prion is shorter or longer than the cellular one.

Single mutations, researchers believe, are also responsible for the species barrier: the fact that prions from one species do not usually infect another. They also determine the length of the incubation period, the duration of the disease, and the type of symptoms.

If a mutation in the prion determines the symptoms in the host, and the symptoms are a direct consequence of the region of the brain that the prions are destroying, it seems to follow that a single mutation is responsible for determining in which area of the brain the prions are going to multiply. How prions could do this is unknown, however.

FROM COWS TO HUMANS

It is generally accepted today that BSE was transmitted and became epidemic among cows as a result of the cannibalistic practice of feeding the processed carcasses of cattle to cows. But how did the BSE prion originate in the first place? Is the BSE agent the scrapie prion that has jumped the species barrier and adapted to cows? Or did the epidemic start with a sporadic case of BSE in a single cow, which was then passed to other cows through their feed?[1] After thorough investigation of the epidemics of the disease, researchers have found data in favor of and against both theories, but no definitive proof. Thus, the origin of the BSE agent may never be known for certain.

Oral transmission of TSE among animals of the same species had already been documented in the 1980s when the BSE epidemic started. Sheep were known to get scrapie by eating contaminated placenta and kuru was reportedly transmitted by the ritualistic eating of the bodies of relatives killed by kuru. Still, the disease had never before jumped the species barrier.

In the 250 years in which scrapie has been known in sheep, not a single case of TSE in cows or humans has been reported in which scrapie was suspected to be the cause. So, when the BSE epidemic started in cows, British authorities were not concerned about the possibility that BSE could be transmitted to humans (or to another species for that matter) by eating contaminated beef. They were wrong. Cases of a new TSE disease eventually appeared in the United Kingdom: in cats starting in 1990, and in humans in the second half of the 1990s. It is accepted today that these cases were directly related to the consumption of BSE-contaminated cows.

The realization that BSE could infect humans caused panic among the British population, who blamed the government for having misled them into believing that beef was safe. The British government responded to the public uproar by issuing strict measures to stop BSE-infected cows from entering the food chain. The specified bovine offal ban of 1989 was followed in December 1995 by a ban forbidding

LOW COST/HIGH PRICE

Eating beef was once the privilege of a wealthy minority. Thanks to the efficiency of today's cattle industry, however, it has become an affordable commodity for just about everyone.

A cow raised grazing freely on pastures takes four to five years to reach the 1,000 pounds it needs to weigh before being slaughtered. But when kept in penned areas where it can barely move and fed corn and protein supplements derived from animal carcasses, the cow reaches the desired weight in less than 18 months.[*]

There is no denying that the rise of the feedlot system has lowered the prices and increased the availability of beef. It has also created an unforeseeable chain of events that culminated in the BSE epidemic in cows and the emergence of the variant form of CJD in humans.

And BSE and vCJD are not the only problems that raising cows in assembly lines has caused. Forcing cows to eat corn—not the food their stomachs have evolved to digest—makes the first of their stomachs' four digestive chambers swell with gas. The gas weakens the stomach walls and allows bacteria to go into the bloodstream and eventually infect the liver. To solve this problem, the cows are given massive doses of antibiotics. But doing this has had a very disturbing effect: the appearance of antibiotic-resistant bacteria. These bacteria are already causing infections in humans that no known antibiotics can treat.

So far, human meddlings have awakened an ancient curse (prion diseases) and created "superbugs" (antibiotic-resistant bacteria). What's next?

[*] *The New York Times Magazine*, March 31, 2002, p. 236.

the slaughterhouses to recover meat mechanically from the vertebrae to prevent contamination with the spinal cord and dorsal root ganglia. On March 1996, cattle older than 30 months were also banned from human food. And for two years (1997 to 1999), the sale of beef on the bone (T-bone steaks and ribs, among others) was also banned in the United Kingdom. Measures were also taken to prevent infected cows from being rendered into cattle food.

The 1988 ban to feed ruminant-derived meat-and-bone meal (MBM) to other ruminants had already been extended in 1994 to include all mammal protein. In 1996, the ban was extended again—this time so that no mammal protein MBM could be used as food for any kind of animals. The government also issued a massive recall on feed from farms and storage sites, and in August 1996, made it illegal even to keep mammalian MBM with other livestock feed.

These measures seem to have been effective. By 2003, in the United Kingdom, only two dozen cows born after August 1996 had been found to be infected with BSE. According to the CDC:

> In the United States, the feeding of rendered cattle products to other cattle has been prohibited since 1997, and the importation of cattle and cattle products from countries with BSE or considered to be at high risk for BSE has been prohibited since 1989; these measures have minimized the potential exposure of animals and humans to the BSE agent.[2]

But are we totally safe?

IS THE MADNESS OVER?

Since the beginning of the 21st century, experts have agreed that to eat beef or drink milk from cows poses no risk of contracting vCJD. Yet offal (waste from butchered animals) should be avoided and is still banned from human consumption. But eating beef is not the only way BSE can be transmitted to humans. Experts also worry about consumer products that might contain bovine material, such as drugs, materials used in transplants, and even leather products. As late as 2001, some pharmaceutical companies were still using parts of cattle that could contain prions (if the cows were infected with BSE) to make nine widely used vaccines, including those for polio, diphtheria, and tetanus. Dietary supplements (especially those that claim to stimulate energy, sexual vitality, and memory) may also contain nervous system, organ, and glandular tissue from cattle. All of these tissues may harbor prions.

Besides the risks of getting vCJD from BSE-infected cows, experts also worry that vCJD might be spread through blood transfusions[3] or organ donations from vCJD-infected donors or by vCJD-contaminated surgical instruments.

Furthermore, BSE is not the only spongiform disease experts are worrying about. If the BSE prion was able to adapt and infect humans, couldn't humans become infected from eating deer or elk infected with chronic wasting disease as well? Or, if the BSE prion were indeed the scrapie prion that has adapted to cows, could it infect sheep and cause a new prion disease in sheep? Could humans then get a new form of TSE from eating sheep infected with the BSE prion?

As of 2002, British epidemiologists estimated that, at most, a few dozen sheep had been contaminated with BSE at that time.[4] This is a very small number out of the almost 40 million sheep that exist in the United Kingdom (Figure 8.1).

DIAGNOSIS OF TSE DISEASES

Cows infected with BSE have been banned from human consumption since the beginning of the BSE epidemic. Yet, because the disease has such a long incubation time, many cows that were already infected but had no symptoms passed unnoticed. The development of a diagnostic test to detect the

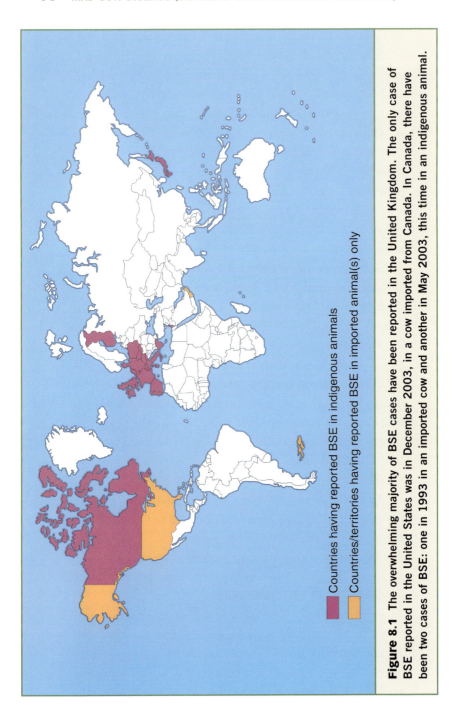

Countries having reported BSE in indigenous animals

Countries/territories having reported BSE in imported animal(s) only

Figure 8.1 The overwhelming majority of BSE cases have been reported in the United Kingdom. The only case of BSE reported in the United States was in December 2003, in a cow imported from Canada. In Canada, there have been two cases of BSE: one in 1993 in an imported cow and another in May 2003, this time in an indigenous animal.

disease while it is still in the incubation period is very much needed.

The only diagnostic test available in the 1980s was to inoculate lab animals with brain samples from cows suspected of having been infected and to wait months—sometimes even longer than a year—to see whether the lab animals came down with the disease. It was not a very efficient test.

Since then, several companies have developed immuno-logical tests that use antibodies to detect pathogenic prions in the brain samples. These tests can be performed in four to six hours. The brain samples from the suspected animals are first digested with proteases to eliminate the cellular prions in both healthy and sick animal brains. Then, they are exposed to the prion-specific antibodies. These antibodies are obtained from laboratory mice that do not have the prion protein.

Because some of the pathogenic prions (PrP^{Sc}) are also digested by proteases, these tests may underestimate the total amount of pathogenic prions. To avoid this problem, in 2002, Prusiner's lab designed a more accurate test that uses anti-bodies specific to certain epitopes (a certain portion of the amino acid sequence) that are hidden in the cellular prion and become exposed when the protein is refolded into the pathogenic conformation.

Although immunological tests are more sensitive, they still require brain samples from the suspected host and thus cannot be done without killing the animal. In the search for a live test, blood and urine samples have been used.

Ruth Gabison at Hadassah University Hospital in Jerusalem found a new version of the PrP^{Sc} in urine samples of scrapie-infected hamsters, BSE cows, and CJD humans.[5] Further research is needed to see if these urinary prions are good indicators of whether an animal has a prion disease.

If prions are present in blood, they are there in such low levels that current tests cannot detect them. A way to avoid this problem would be to increase the amount of PrP^{Sc} in the sample. Several approaches have been tried. The most promising results were obtained in Claudio Soto's lab at Serono Pharmaceutical Research Institute in Geneva. Soto's approach is based on the theory that the lethal prion is a crystal to which the cellular proteins bind. The idea was to blast the samples with ultrasound waves (sonication) before adding brain samples of healthy animals as the source of cellular prion protein. This process, Soto hoped, would break the pathogenic prion crystals and increase the number of seeds to which the prion cellular protein could bind. In the June 14, 2001, issue of *Nature*, Soto's team reported a 60-fold increase in the prion content in their samples after several steps of sonication followed by incubation with a source of cellular prion.[6] A kit for prion detection in blood may follow.

The fact that successive sonication and incubation steps increase the amount of prion protein is evidence in favor of the crystallization theory as the way that the cellular prion becomes pathogenic. This method could also help settle the argument of whether prions are really the agent that causes TSE. Sonication/incubation of a sample containing cellular prions and traces of the pathogenic prion could produce enough new pathogenic prions to cause TSE in healthy animals after inoculation. Experiments in this direction are under way.

FUTURE TREATMENT OF TSE DISEASES

TSE diseases have been known for hundreds of years in the case of scrapie and almost a hundred years in the case of CJD, but no cure has yet been found, although not for lack of trying. Using different approaches, many research teams have been looking for drugs that might be able to destroy the pathogenic prions.

Some teams base their search on the molecular knowledge available about prions and target the drugs to specific steps in the disease. They try, for instance, to prevent PrP^{Sc} from reaching the brain, to prevent the binding of the pathogenic prion outside the cell to the cellular prion sitting on the cell membrane, to prevent the interaction of cellular prion protein and protein X, or to prevent the conversion of the normal prion into pathogenic configuration. Although promising results have been obtained in some of these areas, more research is still needed.

Other scientists, such as Byron Caughey at the Rocky Mountain Laboratories of the National Institutes of Health (NIH), argue that it is not necessary to know how the drug works, as long as it *does* work. They advocate the shotgun approach. This approach aims to generate thousands of compounds and screen them for their ability to destroy prions in vitro. The ones that work are consequently tested on cultured cells and then in vivo in laboratory animals.

Carsten Korth, working at the University of California at San Francisco in 2001, tried another approach. Instead of looking for new drugs, he decided to try the drugs that had already been used in the treatment of other neurological diseases. After all, he thought, these drugs had been proven to be able to reach the brain. One of them, chlorpromazine, had the expected effect of destroying prions in cell cultures. But it wasn't perfect; even after one week of treatment, some prions remained.

Prusiner advised Korth to check for similar compounds. That is how Korth found quinacrine, a drug used in the treatment of malaria. The drug worked in vitro, destroying prions in mice cell cultures at one-tenth the chlorpromazine dose.[7] Encouraged by these results, they administered the drug to two vCJD patients. Although the cognitive abilities of the patients improved somewhat, the improvement was short-lived and the patients ultimately died. The search has continued. By the end of 2002, Prusiner's team alone had synthesized some 10,000 compounds based on quinacrine.

Looking further into the future, an alternative approach to drugs would be to alter the cellular prion protein in a way that could not be converted to the lethal configuration. This requires genetic manipulation of the prion gene. Mice have already been produced in the laboratory that lack the prion gene. These mice were indeed resistant to prion infection—the pathogenic prion has no protein to convert—but researchers worry about the unknown effects that not having the prion protein might have on the normal development of the animals.

Genetic manipulation of the prion gene seems to be a promising approach to breed prion disease–resistant livestock. Yet it doesn't seem a likely alternative for human therapy.

The use of stem cells as a treatment for prion diseases is another tantalizing possibility because stem cells have the potential to turn into any tissue. (Stem cells are unspecialized cells that have the potential to develop into any kind of cell the body needs.) Preliminary results from experiments done in Great Britain suggest that grafting stem cells into the brains of mice reduces the number of neurons lost after a prion infection. Because stem cell research is presently restricted in the United States, advances in this area must come mainly from other countries.

PREVENTION OF TSE DISEASES

Rather than fighting the prion with an outside drug, it might be more effective to help the body do its own fighting. This is the idea behind a virus vaccine: to stimulate the body's immune system to produce antibodies against the virus by inoculating a portion of the virus or a dead virus. Later, when the body is infected with the real virus, these specific antibodies will bind to it and destroy it, stopping the spread of the disease.

But researchers fear that a vaccine against prions would not be feasible because prions do not elicit an immune response in the body. Because prions are cellular proteins, the body does not recognize them as foreign molecules and does not produce antibodies against them. Even if the body were to produce antibodies against prions, these antibodies would be likely to recognize their own cellular prion proteins and destroy them. Despite all these concerns, the following results suggest that a prion vaccine might still be possible.

At the University of Zurich, Frank L. Heppner, Adriano Aguzzi, and their colleagues created mice genetically engineered to produce antibodies against the prion protein.[8] After being inoculated with the pathogenic prion, the animals remained healthy. What's more, these mice didn't show any immune response against their own prions.

Scientists are investigating new ways to induce an immune response against the prion in wild-type mice. Promising results have been obtained by using either modified versions of the prion protein or by combining it with either virus-like particles or antibodies.

Successful therapy against prion diseases is still in the future. But the spectacular advances seen in the field, in the last few years, at least, give us hope that is possible to fight back against BSE and other diseases.

Glossary

Amino acids—The basic building blocks of proteins. The body makes many amino acids. Others come from food and the body breaks them down for use by cells.

Amyloid plaques—Waxy translucent substances consisting of protein in combination with polysaccharides that are deposited in some animal organs and tissue under abnormal conditions (such as in Alzheimer's disease).

Cerebellum—The part of the human brain between the brain stem and the back of the cerebrum; it controls balance and movement.

Cerebral cortex—A 1/8-inch-thick gray outer layer of the human brain that controls higher mental functions.

Chromosome—Microscopic structure within cells that carries the molecule deoxyribonucleic acid (DNA), the hereditary material that influences the development and characteristics of each organism.

Chronic wasting disease (**CWD**)—The only transmissible spongiform encephalopathy (TSE) currently found in free-ranging wildlife, such as white-tailed deer, mule deer, and elk. It has also been found in captive animals of similar species.

Electroencephalograms—Tests that register brain waves.

Fatal familial insomnia (**FFI**)—A hereditary disease. Its most characteristic symptoms are insomnia, hallucinations, dream enactments, and twitching.

Floral or **florid plaques**—Plaques surrounded by a circle of vacuoles that makes them look like a flower.

Gerstmann-Sträussler-Scheinker syndrome (**GSS**)—An inheritable form of transmissible spongiform encephalopathy (TSE) in humans.

Glia—The major support cells of the brain; they support and protect the neurons.

Greaves—A product of the rendering process, it is produced when the heavier protein sinks to the bottom.

Hormones—Chemical messengers that play an essential role in the development of the human body and are responsible for the development of secondary sexual characteristics.

Iatrogenic transmission—The accidental spread of a disease in a medical setting.

Ionizing radiation—Electromagnetic radiation whose waves contain enough energy to overcome the binding energy of electrons in atoms or molecules, thus creating ions.

Kuru—A degenerative nerve disease caused by a prion (infectious protein) transmitted to humans via contaminated human brain tissue.

Louping ill or **loup**—A disease in sheep caused by a tick-borne virus that induces brain damage.

Meat-and-bone meal (MBM)—A protein-rich food to accelerate growth and increase milk production in cows.

Mutations—Accidental changes that occur when a DNA gene is damaged or changed in such a way as to alter the genetic message carried by that gene.

Neurons—The functional cells of the brain that carry information between the brain and other parts of the body.

Nucleotides—The individual units that make up DNA. Each nucleotide has a sugar, a phosphate, and a base.

Placenta—The organ that unites mother and offspring during pregnancy and is expelled at birth. It provides nourishment and a means for the offspring to eliminate waste.

Prion—A protein particle that is capable of causing infection or disease. Similar to a virus, it is not capable of reproduction by itself. Unlike a virus, it does not contain genetic material (DNA or RNA).

Proteases—Active proteins or enzymes that are found in all cells and destroy other proteins. They are enzymes that specifically digest proteins by breaking the bonds between amino acids.

Purifying—Separating one agent from other components in order to remove contaminants.

Rendering—Boiling animal carcasses to separate the fat from the meat.

Ruminants—Hoofed mammals that chew their cud and usually have a four-chambered stomach, like cows, sheep, and oxen.

Scrapie—A fatal nervous system disorder that has affected sheep in England for over 250 years. It is characterized by chronic itching, loss of muscular control, and progressive degeneration of the central nervous system.

Tallow—A product of the rendering process, it is fat that separates and floats as a creamy white substance.

Glossary

Transmissible mink encephalopathy (**TME**)—A very rare disease of ranch-reared mink that, when it occurs, can have a mortality rate as high as 100 percent of the breeding animals.

tRNA—Transfer RNA, or amino acid transporters.

Vacuoles—Large membrane-bound compartments within some cells that serve the following functions: capturing food materials or unwanted structural debris surrounding the cell, capturing materials that might be toxic to the cell, maintaining fluid balance within the cell, exporting unwanted substances from the cell, or determining relative cell size.

Virino—A very small virus without a protein coat, thought to be the cause of scrapie and other degenerative diseases of the central nervous system.

Viroids—Plant viruses that are only very small bits of RNA. Viroids are about one-tenth the size of the smallest virus known to date.

Virus—A strand of nucleic acid inside a coat of proteins. It is a cause of various important diseases in humans, animals, and plants.

Notes

CHAPTER 1:
MAD COW DISEASE: THE BEGINNING

1 Maxime Schwartz, *How the Cows Turned Mad.* Berkeley, CA: University of California Press, 2003, p. 143.

2 Raymond Bradley, "Memo of December 19, 1986," evidence for Report of the BSE Inquiry. London: Her Majesty's Stationery Office, 2000, as quoted in Philip Yam, *The Pathological Protein: Mad Cow, Chronic Wasting, and Other Deadly Prion Diseases.* New York: Springer-Verlag, 2003, p. 109.

3 Yam, p. 113.

4 Schwartz, p. 150.

5 Richard Rhodes, *Deadly Feasts.* New York: Simon & Schuster, 1997, p. 180.

6 Gabriel Horn, et al., "Review of the Origin of BSE, July 5, 2001." London: Department for Food, Environment and Rural Affairs, 2001, p. 15, as quoted in Philip Yam, *The Pathological Protein*, pp. 115–116.

7 Rhodes, p. 177.

8 Schwartz, p. 144.

9 Yam, p. 114.

10 Ibid., p. 116.

11 Ibid., pp. 114–115.

12 Schwartz, p. 149.

13 Ibid., p. 150.

CHAPTER 2:
vCJD: THE HUMAN BSE

1 "The Southwood Working Party, 1988–89." Report of the BSE Inquiry, vol. 4. London: Her Majesty's Stationery Office, 2000, as quoted in Philip Yam, *The Pathological Protein: Mad Cow, Chronic Wasting, and Other Deadly Prion Diseases.* New York: Springer-Verlag, 2003, p. 118.

2 Yam, p. 120.

3 Richard Rhodes, *Deadly Feasts.* New York: Simon & Schuster 1997, p. 182.

4 Ibid., p. 185.

5 T. A. Holt and J. Philips, "Bovine Spongiform Encephalopathy," *British Medical Journal*, vol. 296, June 4, 1988, pp. 1581–1582, as quoted in Maxime Schwartz, *How the Cows Turned Mad.* Berkeley, CA: University of California Press, 2003, p. 153.

6 R. G. Will, J. W. Ironside, and M. Zeidler, et al., "A New Variant of Creutzfeldt-Jakob Disease in the UK." *The Lancet* 347 (1996): 921–925.

7 Madeline Drexler, *Secret Agents: The Menace of Emerging Infections.* Washington, D.C.: Joseph Henry Press, 2002, p. 95.

8 Available online at *http://www.dh.gov.uk/ PublicationsAndStatistics/PressReleases/ PressReleasesNotices/fs/en?CONTENT_ID =4083581&chk=QYhSNS.*

CHAPTER 3:
SPONGIFORM ENCEPHALOPATHIES IN HUMANS

1 S. J. DeArmond and J. W. Ironsides, "Neuropathology of Prion Diseases," in Stanley B. Prusiner, ed., *Prion Biology and Diseases.* Cold Spring Harbor, NY: Cold Spring Harbor Laboratory Press, 1999, pp. 585–652; Philip Yam, *The Pathological Protein: Mad Cow, Chronic Wasting, and Other Deadly Prion Diseases.* New York: Springer-Verlag, 2003, p. 20.

2 Richard T. Johnson and Clarence J. Gibbs, Jr., "Creutzfeldt-Jakob Disease and Related Transmissible Spongiform Encephalopathies." *New England Journal of Medicine* 339 (27) (1998): 1994–2004, as quoted in Philip Yam, *The Pathological Protein*, p. 16.

3 Yam, p. 28.

Notes

4 Philip Yam interview with Paul Brown, Bethesda, Maryland, February 27, 2002, as quoted in Philip Yam, *The Pathological Protein*, p. 28.

5 William J. Hadlow, "The Scrapie-Kuru Connection: Recollections of How It Came About," as quoted in Stanley B. Prusiner, ed., *Prion Diseases in Humans and Animals*. New York: Ellis Harwood, 1992, p. 43.

CHAPTER 4:
SCRAPIE AND OTHER SPONGIFORM ENCEPHALOPATHIES IN ANIMALS

1 J. G. Leopold, *Nutzliche und auf die Erfahrung gegrundete Einleitung zu der Landwirthschaft, funf heile.* Berlin, Germany: Christian Friedrich Gunthern, 1759, p. 348; Paul Brown and Raymond Bradley, "1775 and All That: A Historical Primer of Transmissible Spongiform Encephalopathy," *British Medical Journal* 317 (1998): 7174, as quoted in M. J. Walters, *Six Modern Plagues and How We Are Causing Them*. Washington, D.C.: Island Press, 2003, p. 31.

2 Ibid., as quoted in Philip Yam, *The Pathological Protein: Mad Cow, Chronic Wasting, and Other Deadly Prion Diseases*. New York: Springer-Verlag, 2003, p. 38.

3 T. Comber, "Letters to Reader Peacock, Esq., and Dr Hunter, Concerning the Rickets in Sheep." *Real Improvements in Agriculture*. London: Phillips, 1811, pp. 145–146, as cited in Maxime Schwartz, *How the Cows Turned Mad*. Berkeley, CA: University of California Press, 2003, p. 6.

4 Ridley Rosalind and Harry Baker, *Fatal Protein: The Story of CJD, BSE, and Other Prion Diseases*. New York: Oxford University Press, 1998.

5 W. S. Gordon, "Advances in Veterinarian Research: Louping Ill, Tick-Borne Fever and Scrapie." *Veterinary Records* 58 (1946): 516–520, as cited in Maxime Schwartz, *How the Cows Turned Mad*, pp. 42–43.

6 R. F. Marsh and W. J. Hadlow, "Transmissible Mink Encephalopathy." *Scientific and Technical Review* (June 11, 1992), p. 547, as quoted in Philip Yam, *The Pathological Protein*, p. 166.

7 Richard Rhodes, *Deadly Feasts*. New York: Simon & Schuster, 1997, p. 227.

8 E. S. Williams and S. Young, "Chronic Wasting Disease of Captive Mule Deer: A Spongiform Encephalopathy," *Journal of Wildlife Diseases* 16 (1980): 89–98, as quoted in Philip Yam, *The Pathological Protein*, p. 174.

CHAPTER 5:
SPONGIFORM ENCEPHALOPATHIES ARE TRANSMISSABLE

1 C. J. Gibbs, Jr., "Spongiform Encephalopathies—Slow, Latent, and Temperate Virus Infections—in Restrospect," as quoted in Stanley B. Prusiner, ed., *Prion Diseases in Humans and Animals*. New York: Ellis Harwood, 1992, p. 56.

2 D. Carleton Gajdusek, "Kuru in the New Guinea Highlands." *Tropical Neurology*. London: Oxford University Press, 1973, p. 382, as quoted in Philip Yam, *The Pathological Protein*, p. 48.

3 Maxime Schwartz, *How the Cows Turned Mad*. Berkeley, CA: University of California Press, 2003, p. 46.

4 Philip Yam, *The Pathological Protein: Mad Cow, Chronic Wasting, and Other Deadly Prion Diseases*. New York: Springer-Verlag, 2003, p. 82.

CHAPTER 6:
FROM SLOW VIRUS TO PRIONS

1 Tikvah Alper, "Photo- and Radiobiology of the Scrapie Agent," in Stanley Prusiner, ed., *Prion Disease of Humans and Animals.* New York: Ellis Harwood, 1992, p. 31.

2 T. Alper, W. A. Cramp, D. A. Haig, and M. C. Clarke, "Does the Agent of Scrapie Replicate Without Nucleic Acid?" *Nature* 214 (1967): 764–766.

3 James Watson and Francis Crick, "A Structure for Deoxyribose Nucleic Acid." *Nature* 171 (1953): 737. Available online at *http://biocrs.biomed .brown.edu/Books/Chapters/Ch%208/ DH-Paper.html.*

4 James Watson, *The Double Helix.* New York: W.W. Norton, 1981.

5 Richard Rhodes, *Deadly Feasts.* New York: Simon & Schuster, 1997, p. 119.

6 Autobiography of Stanley B. Prusiner, Nobel Prize.org. Available online at *http://www.nobel.se/medicine/ laureates/1997/prusiner-autobio .html.*

7 G. Taubes, "The Name of the Game Is Fame, But Is It Science? Stanley Prusiner, 'Discoverer' of Prions," *Discover* (December 1986), pp. 28–52, as quoted in Philip Yam, *The Pathological Protein,* p. 61.

8 Stanley B. Prusiner, "Novel Proteinaceous Infectious Particles Cause Scrapie," *Science* 216 (1982): 136–144, as quoted in Maxime Schwartz, *How the Cows Turned Mad,* p. 100.

9 Philip Yam, *The Pathological Protein: Mad Cow, Chronic Wasting, and Other Deadly Prion Diseases.* New York: Springer-Verlag, 2003, p. 83.

CHAPTER 7:
MORE ON PRIONS

1 Stanley B. Prusiner, "Development of the Prion Concept." *Prion Biology and Diseases.* Cold Spring Harbor, NY: Cold Spring Harbor Laboratory Press, 1999, p. 93.

2 P. A. Merz, et al., "Abnormal Fibrils from Scrapie-Infected Brain." *Acta Neuropathologica* 54 (1981): 63.

3 B. Oesch, et al., "A Cellular Gene Encodes Scrapie PrP 27–30 Protein," *Cell* 40 (1985): 735.

4 B. Chesebro, et al., "A Cellular Gene Encodes Scrapie Prion Protein— Specific mRNA in Scrapie-Infected and Uninfected Brain." *Nature* 315 (1985): 331.

5 Maxime Schwartz, *How the Cows Turned Mad.* Berkeley, CA: University of California Press, 2003, p. 112.

6 Stanley B. Prusiner, "Prion Diseases." *Scientific American* (January 1995): 51, as quoted in Philip Yam, *The Pathological Protein,* p. 71.

7 Ibid., as quoted in Yam, p. 72.

8 Philip Yam, interview with Charles Weissmann, *The Pathological Protein: Mad Cow, Chronic Wasting, and Other Deadly Prion Diseases.* New York: Springer-Verlag, 2003, p. 95.

9 Ibid., p. 98.

10 Review of the Origin of BSE. Available online at *http://www.defra.gov.uk/ animalh/bse/bseorigin.pdf.*

CHAPTER 8:
MAD COW DISEASE REVISITED

1 Department of Health and Human Services, Centers for Disease Control and Prevention, "Bovine Spongiform Encephalopathy in a Dairy Cow— Washington State 2003." *Morbidity and Mortality Weekly Report*

Notes

(January 9, 2004), vols. 52, 53, pp. 1280–1285. Available online at *http://www.cdc.gov/mmwr/preview/ mmwrhtml/mm5253a2.htm.*

2 Scott A. Norton, "Raw Animal Tissues and Dietary Supplements." *New England Journal of Medicine* 343 (2000): 304–305.

3 Philip Yam, interview with Robert G. Will, Edinburgh, Scotland, October 31, 2001.

4 R. R. Kao, M. B. Gravenor, M. Baylis, et al. "The Potential Size and Duration of an Epidemic of Bovine Spongiform Encephalopathy in British Sheep." *Science* 295 (2002): 332–335.

5 G. M. Shaked, Y. Shaked, and Z. Kariv-Inbal, et al. "A Protease-Resistant Prion Protein Isoform Is Present in Urine of Animals and Humans Affected with Prion Diseases." *Journal of Biological Chemistry* 276 (2001): 31479–31482.

6 G. P. Saborio, B. Permanne, and C. Soto. "Sensitive Detection of Pathological Prion Protein by Cyclic Amplification of Protein Misfolding." *Nature* 412 (2001): 739–743.

7 C. Korth, B.C.H. May, and F. E. Cohen, et al. "Acridine and Phenotiazine Derivatives as Pharmacotherapeutics for Prion Disease" *Proceedings of the National Academy of Sciences of the United States of America* 98 (2001): 9836–9841.

8 F. L. Heppner, C. Musahl, and I. Arrighi, et al. "Prevention of Scrapie Pathogenesis by Transgenic Expression of Anti-Prion Protein Antibodies." *Science* 294 (2001): 178–182; F. L. Heppner, I. Arrighi, and U. Kalinke, et al. "Immunity against Prions?" *Trends in Molecular Medicine* 7 (2001): 477–479.

Bibliography

BOOKS AND ARTICLES

Alberts, B., D. Bray, J. Lewis, M. Raff, K. Roberts, and J. D. Watson. *Molecular Biology of the Cell*, 3rd ed. New York: Garland Publishing, 1994.

Alper, T., W. A. Cramp, D. A. Haig, and M. C. Clarke. "Does the Agent of Scrapie Replicate Without Nucleic Acid?" *Nature* 214 (1967): 764–766.

Belay, E. D., and L. B. Schonberger. "Variant Creutzfeldt-Jakob Disease and Bovine Spongiform Encephalopathy." *Clinical Laboratory Medicine* 22 (2002): 849–862.

Brown, P., and R. Bradley. "1775 and All That: A Historical Primer of Transmissible Spongiform Encephalopathy." *British Medical Journal* 317 (1998): 1688–1692.

Brown, P., R. G. Will, R. Bradley, D. M. Asher, and L. Detwiler. "Bovine Spongiform Encephalopathy and Variant Creutzfeldt-Jakob Disease: Background, Evolution, and Current Concerns." *Emerging Infectious Diseases* 7 (2001): 6–16.

Chesebro, B., et al. "A Cellular Gene Encodes Scrapie Prion Protein—Specific mRNA in Scrapie-Infected and Uninfected Brain." *Nature* 315 (1985): 331.

Collinge, J., and M. S. Palmer, eds. *Prion Diseases*. New York: Oxford University Press, 1997.

Court, L., and B. Dodet, eds. *Transmissible Subacute Spongiform Encephalopathies: Prion Diseases*. Paris: Elsevier, 1998.

Dealler, S. *Lethal Legacy: BSE—The Search for the Truth*. London: Bloomsbury, 1996.

Drexler, M. *Secret Agents: The Menace of Emerging Infections*. Washington, D.C.: Joseph Henry Press, 2002.

Gajdusek, D. Carleton. "Kuru in the New Guinea Highlands." *Tropical Neurology*. London: Oxford University Press, 1973.

Gibbons, R. V., R. C. Holman, E. D. Belay, and L. B. Schonberger. "Creutzfeldt-Jakob disease in the United States: 1979–1998." *Journal of the American Medical Association* 284 (2000): 2322–2323.

Hadlow, W. J. *The Scrapie-Kuru Connection: Recollections of How It Came About, in Prion Diseases in Humans and Animals*, ed. Stanley B. Prusiner, et al. New York: Ellis Harwood, 1992, p. 43.

Heppner, F. L., I. Arrighi, U. Kalinke, et al. "Immunity against Prions?" *Trends in Molecular Medicine* 7 (2001): 477–479.

Bibliography

Heppner, F. L., C. Musahl, I. Arrighi, et al. "Prevention of Scrapie Pathogenesis by Transgenic Expression of Anti-Prion Protein Antibodies." *Science* 294 (2001): 178–182.

Holt, T. A., and J. Philips. "Bovine Spongiform Encephalopathy." *British Medical Journal* 296 (1988): 1581–1582.

Johnson, R. T., and C. J. Gibbs, Jr. "Creutzfeldt-Jakob Disease and Related Transmissible Spongiform Encephalopathies." *New England Journal of Medicine* 339 (1998): 1994–2004.

Kao, R. R., M. B. Gravenor, M. Baylis, et al. "The Potential Size and Duration of an Epidemic of Bovine Spongiform Encephalopathy in British Sheep." *Science* 295 (2002): 332–335.

Klitzman, R. *The Trembling Mountain. A Personal Account of Kuru, Cannibals and Mad Cow Disease.* New York: Plenum Trade, 1998.

Korth, C., B.C.H. May, F. E. Cohen, et al. "Acridine and Phenothiazine Derivatives as Pharmacotherapeutics for Prion Disease." *Proceedings of the National Academy of Sciences of the United States of America* 98 (2001): 9836–9841.

Marsh, R. F., and W. J. Hadlow. "Transmissible Mink Encephalopathy." *Scientific and Technical Review* (1992): 547.

Merz, P. A., et al. "Abnormal Fibrils from Scrapie-Infected Brain." *Acta Neuropathologica* 54 (1981): 63.

Norton, Scott A. "Raw Animal Tissues and Dietary Supplements." *New England Journal of Medicine* 343 (2000): 304–305.

Oesch, B., et al. "A Cellular Gene Encodes Scrapie PrP 27-30 Protein." *Cell* 40 (1985): 735.

Prusiner, S. B. "Novel Proteinaceous Infectious Particles Cause Scrapie." *Science* 216 (1982): 136–144.

———. *Prion Biology and Diseases,* ed. Stanley B. Prusiner. Cold Spring Harbor, NY: Cold Spring Harbor Laboratory Press, 1999.

———. "The Prion Diseases." *Scientific American,* January 1995: 51.

———, ed. *Prions Prions Prions.* Berlin and Heidelberg: Springer-Verlag, 1996.

Rampton, S., and J. C. Stauber. *Mad Cow USA: Could the Nightmare Happen Here?* Monroe, ME: Common Courage Press, 1997.

Ratzan, S. C. *The Mad Cow Crisis, Health and the Public Good.* London: UCL Press, 1998.

Rhodes, R. *Deadly Feasts.* New York: Simon & Schuster, 1997.

Ridley, R. M., and H. F. Baker. *Fatal Protein: The Story of CJD, BSE, and Other Prion Diseases.* New York: Oxford University Press, 1998.

Rohwer, R. "The Scrapie Agent: 'A Virus by Any Other Name.'" *Current Topics in Microbiology and Immunology* 172 (1991): 195–232.

Saborio, G. P., B. Permanne, and C. Soto. "Sensitive Detection of Pathological Prion Protein by Cyclic Amplification of Protein Misfolding." *Nature* 412 (2001): 739–743.

Schwartz, M. *How the Cows Turned Mad.* Berkeley, CA: University of California Press, 2003.

Shaked, G. M., Y. Shaked, Z. Kariv-Inbal, et al. "A Protease-Resistant Prion Protein Isoform Is Present in Urine of Animals and Humans Affected with Prion Diseases." *Journal of Biological Chemistry* 276 (2001): 31479–31482.

Taubes, G. "The Name of the Game Is Fame. But Is It Science? Stanley Prusiner, 'Discoverer' of Prions." *Discover* (December 1986): 28–52.

Talaro, K., and A. Talaro. *Foundations in Microbiology.* New York: W. C. Brown Publishers, 1993.

Vonnegut, Kurt. *Cat's Cradle.* New York: Bantam Doubleday Dell Publishing Group, Inc., 1998.

Wallace, R. A. *Biology: The World of Life*, 6th ed. New York: Harper Collins Publishers, 1992.

Walters, M. J. *Six Modern Plagues and How We Are Causing Them.* Washington, D.C.: Island Press, 2003.

Watson, J. D. *The Double Helix*, ed. G. S. Stent. New York: W. W. Norton, 1981.

Watson, J. D., and F.H.C. Crick. "Molecular Structure of Nucleic Acids: A Structure for Deoxyribose Nucleic Acid." *Nature* 171 (1953): 737. Available online at *http://biocrs.biomed.brown.edu/Books/Chapters/Ch%208/ DH-Paper.html.*

Will, R. G., J. W. Ironside, M. Zeidler, et al. "A New Variant of Creutzfeldt-Jakob Disease in the UK." *The Lancet* 347 (1996): 921–925.

Will, R., M. Zeidler, and G. E. Stewart. "Diagnosis of New Variant Creutzfeldt-Jakob Disease." *Annals of Neurology* 47 (2000): 575–582.

Bibliography

Williams, E. S., and S. Young. "Chronic Wasting Disease of Captive Mule Deer: A Spongiform Encephalopathy." *Journal of Wildlife Diseases* 16 (1980): 89–98.

Wolfe, S. L. *Introduction to Cell and Molecular Biology.* Wadsworth Publishing Company, 1995.

Yam, P. *The Pathological Protein: Mad Cow, Chronic Wasting and Other Deadly Prion Disease.* New York: Springer-Verlag, 2003.

Zigas, V. *Laughing Death: The Untold Story of Kuru.* Clifton, NJ: Humana Press, 1990.

Further Reading

BOOKS AND MAGAZINES

Collinge, J., and M. S. Palmer, eds. *Prion Diseases.* New York: Oxford University Press, 1997.

Drexler, M. *Secret Agents: The Menace of Emerging Infections.* Washington, D.C.: Joseph Henry Press, 2002.

Prusiner, S. B. "The Prion Diseases." *Scientific American* (January 1995).

Rhodes, R. *Deadly Feasts.* New York: Simon & Schuster, 1997.

Ridgway, Tom. *Mad Cow Disease: Bovine Spongiform Encephalopathy.* New York: Rosen, 2002.

Schwartz, M. *How the Cows Turned Mad.* Berkeley, CA: University of California Press, 2003.

Sheen, Barbara. *Mad Cow Disease.* San Diego: Lucent Books, 2004.

VIDEO

The Brain Eater: Mad Cow Disease
NOVA. Celebrating 20 years. 1998.
Produced by Bettina Lerner & Joseph McMasters
Exec. Producer Paula S. Apsell
BBC TV/WGBH Boston co-production
Copyright 1998. WGBH Educational Foundation

Websites

Animal and Plant Health Inspection Service, USDA
http://www.aphis.usda.gov/lpa/issues/issues.html

Centers for Disease Control and Prevention (CDC)
http://www.cdc.gov/ncidod/diseases/cjd/cjd.htm

Chronic Wasting Disease Alliance
http://www.cwd-info.org/

CJD Foundation
http://www.cjdfoundation.org/

CJD Voice
http://members.aol.com/larmstr853/cjdvoice/index.htm

Food and Drug Administration
http://www.fda.gov/cber/bse/bse.htm

Human BSE foundation
http://www.hbsef.org/

MedicineNet.com
http://www.medicinenet.com/script/main/hp.asp

National Library of Medicine
http://www.nlm.nih.gov/

Organic Consumer Association on Mad Cow Disease
http://organicconsumers.org/madcow.htm

Priondata.org
http://www.priondata.org/

The U.K. Creutzfeldt-Jakob Disease Surveillance Unit
http://www.cjd.ed.ac.uk/

U.K. Department for Environment, Food and Rural Affairs
http://www.defra.gov.uk/

Index

Picture Credits

10: Public Health Image Library (PHIL), Courtesy CDC
16: PHIL, Courtesy CDC
20: Information from the OIE, World Organisation for Animal Health
22: Associated Press, AP/Jim James
24: Information from *Emerging Infectious Diseases,* © Peter Lamb
29: © MC PHERSON COLIN/CORBIS SYGMA
31: © Science VU/Visuals Unlimited
35: Courtesy of the National CJD Surveillance Unit, Western General Hospital, Edinburgh
36: United Nations Cartography Section, Map No. 4104 Rev. 1
50: © Dr. Terry Kreeger/Visuals Unlimited

59: © Peter Lamb
62: © Peter Lamb
63: © Peter Lamb
66: © Peter Lamb
68: Associated Press, AP/Markus Schreiber
69: © Peter Lamb
72: © Peter Lamb
75: © Peter Lamb
79: © Peter Lamb
80: © Stanley B. Prusiner/Visuals Unlimited
87: © Peter Lamb
98: © Peter Lamb, recreated by permission of the World Organisation for Animal Health (OIE)

Cover: © VAN PARYS/CORBIS SYGMA

About the Author

A native of Spain, **Carmen Ferreiro** obtained her doctoral degree in biology from the Universidad Autónoma of Madrid. She worked as a researcher for over 10 years in Spain and at the University of California at Davis and has published several papers in the biochemistry and molecular biology fields. She has also written books on *Heroin* and *Ritalin* for the Chelsea House series DRUGS: THE STRAIGHT FACTS. She lives in Pennsylvania as an independent writer and translator.

About the Editor

The late **I. Edward Alcamo** was a Distinguished Teaching Professor of Microbiology at the State University of New York at Farmingdale. Alcamo studied biology at Iona College in New York and earned his M.S. and Ph.D. degrees in microbiology at St. John's University, also in New York. He had taught at Farmingdale for over 30 years. In 2000, Alcamo won the Carski Award for Distinguished Teaching in Microbiology, the highest honor for microbiology teachers in the United States. He was a member of the American Society for Microbiology, the National Association of Biology Teachers, and the American Medical Writers Association. Alcamo authored numerous books on the subjects of microbiology, AIDS, and DNA technology as well as the award-winning textbook *Fundamentals of Microbiology*, now in its sixth edition.